Focused History Taking for OSCEs

A compr...

Foundation Year One Doctor
University Hospital of South Manchester Foundation Trust

GRAHAM McCOLLUM
MB BS BSc
Foundation Year One Doctor
Hull & East Yorkshire Hospitals NHS Trust

PRIHA SHUKLA
MB ChB
Foundation Year Two Doctor
University Hospital of South Manchester/
The Christie NHS Foundation Trusts

PETER McCOLLUM
MB BCh MA MCh FRCSI FRCSEd
Professor of Vascular Surgery
Honorary Consultant Vascular Surgeon
Hull York Medical School/Hull & East Yorkshire
Hospitals NHS Trust

Forewords by

ANTHONY FREEMONT
Head, Undergraduate Medical Education
Professor of Osteoarticular Pathology
University of Manchester

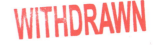

DAVID PEARSON
Deputy Dean (Education)
Hull York Medical School

Radcliffe Publishing
London • New York

Radcliffe Publishing Ltd
St Marks House
Shepherdess Walk
London
N1 7BQ
United Kingdom

www.radcliffehealth.com

Every effort has been made to ensure that the information in this book is accurate. This does not diminish the requirement to exercise clinical judgement, and neither the publisher nor the authors can accept any responsibility for its use in practice.

New research and clinical experience can result in changes in treatment and drug therapy. Users of the information in this book should therefore check the most recent product information on any drug they may prescribe to ensure they are complying with the manufacturer's recommendations concerning dosage, the method and duration of administration and contraindications.

British Library Cataloguing in Publication Data

A catalogue record for this book is available from the British Library.

ISBN-13: 978 184619 581 5

The paper used for the text pages of this book is FSC® certified. FSC (The Forest Stewardship Council®) is an international network to promote responsible management of the world's forests.

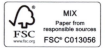

MIX
Paper from
responsible sources
FSC® C013056

Typeset by Darkriver Design, Auckland, New Zealand
Printed and bound by TJI Digital, Padstow, Cornwall, UK

Contents

Foreword by Anthony Freemont   vi
Foreword by David Pearson   vii
Preface   viii
About the authors   ix
Acknowledgements   x
List of abbreviations   xi

Taking a focused history in OSCEs   **1**

General OSCE tips   **7**

Tips for approaching a history-taking OSCE station   **11**

General medicine   **13**
Pain   14
Tiredness   16
Fever   20
Rash   24
Bruising   28

Surgery   **33**
Abdominal pain   34
Lumps, bumps and swellings   38
Weight loss   41
Jaundice   44
Claudication   47

Cardiorespiratory medicine   **51**
Chest pain   52
Breathlessness   56
Palpitations   60

Cough 63
Haemoptysis 66

Gastroenterology 69

Dysphagia 70
Haematemesis 74
Change in bowel habit (constipation/diarrhoea in adults) 78
Bleeding per rectum 82

Renal medicine & urology 87

Haematuria 88
Dysuria 92
Polyuria 96

Neurology 101

Falls 102
Headache 106
Weakness 110
Numbness/paraesthesia 114
Dizziness 118
Hearing loss 121

Psychiatry 125

Low mood/depression 126
Anxiety 129
Hallucinations/delusions 133
Forgetfulness 136
Mania 140
Alcohol history 144
Eating disorder 147
Self-harm/suicide attempt (risk assessment) 150

Obstetrics & gynaecology 153

Gynaecological history template 154
Vaginal bleeding 156
Antepartum haemorrhage 160
Vaginal discharge 163
Subfertility 166
Urinary incontinence 169
Amenorrhoea/oligomenorrhoea 172

Paediatrics 177

Paediatric history template 178

Vomiting   180
Failure to thrive   183
Convulsions   187
Developmental delay   191
Cough   195
Behaviour   198

Musculoskeletal medicine   **201**
Back pain   202
Joint pain   206

Ophthalmology   **211**
Painful red eye   212
Loss of vision/blurry vision   216

Index   221

Foreword by Anthony Freemont

The OSCE examination or its equivalent is rapidly becoming the gold standard in how the clinical knowledge, acumen and skills of undergraduate medical students and postgraduate medical trainees are tested in a controlled and reproducible clinical environment.

In Manchester at any one time, we have in excess of 2200 medical students. Our programme is specifically designed to train students to be independent learners and to set them up for life as doctors in the rapidly changing world of modern medicine and healthcare.

For a student, this book is a perfect learning resource for approaching a whole series of clinical problems. But it goes further, eloquently showing how to construct a successful approach to any clinical problem. I thoroughly recommend this book to all clinical students. If you read it, you will learn a great deal about specific medical problems, see how to approach common clinical scenarios and, perhaps more importantly, learn how to analyse a clinical setting and efficiently extract the information necessary for diagnosis and the initiation of management.

This really is a super little book that goes further than just showing how to pass an exam, but rather equipping the reader with a philosophical approach to any clinical problem. Congratulations to all the authors, but especially David McCollum, who as a fifth-year medical student at Manchester was the life force behind this book.

Professor Anthony Freemont
Head, Undergraduate Medical Education
Professor of Osteoarticular Pathology
University of Manchester
September 2012

Foreword by David Pearson

I am delighted to endorse/write a foreword for this excellent new book on how to approach OSCEs, which involves taking a history and planning patient management. This new book has the great strength of being written by three recent UK medical graduates who have been exposed to a range of OSCEs within their respective medical schools. They have written a practical hands-on guide which supports students in their approach to history taking which will benefit them both in passing OSCEs and once they graduate as a doctor. Medical schools increasingly are using OSCEs as a reliable and safe way to assess their students at all levels of experience. This book will both share advice on how to pass these OSCEs, but will teach skills and approaches of benefit within other clinical examinations and during clinical practice. The various chapters take a structured and clearly laid out approach to common presentations and clinical scenarios, and offer a guide to the essential components of history taking but also cover red flags, investigations and management points.

This book will prove a valuable asset to improve your skills in approaching and assessing patients, and will help pass OSCEs involving history taking and management plans.

Dr David Pearson EdD FRCGP FHEA
Deputy Dean (Education)
Hull York Medical School
September 2012

Preface

Modern-day assessments of medical students place a strong emphasis on the importance of examinations under simulated clinical settings, in which communication skills are becoming a fundamental component of the assessment.

This book is a comprehensive guide to history taking to suit modern medical student examination purposes. The introductory chapter tackles how to construct histories and approach history-based OSCE stations. This includes tips from recently qualified doctors and a highly respected surgeon who commonly examines OSCEs at various levels. This book provides a database of histories based on common presenting complaints in student examinations across the United Kingdom. The histories are based on what you as the student are required to consider and are concisely written with mnemonics provided to aid recall.

In examinations, at the end of each OSCE station the examiner will often ask the student for a differential diagnosis and management plan. At the end of every history, we provide a breakdown of key aspects for differential diagnoses, as well as a list of pertinent investigations and management options.

David McCollum
September 2012

About the authors

Dr David McCollum

David graduated from the University of Manchester's School of Medicine in July 2012 with an MB ChB. He now works as a foundation year one doctor at the University Hospital of South Manchester. His medical interests lie in the field of rheumatology. He travelled to India under sponsorship by Arthritis Research UK to experience rheumatology in India and is currently involved in ongoing research projects with the staff at the Kellgren Centre for Rheumatology, Manchester Royal Infirmary. He has presented at various national and international conferences.

Dr Graham McCollum

Graham graduated from Hull/York Medical School in July 2012 with an MB BS BSc. David and Graham are twins. Graham intercalated in human physiology at the University of Leeds in 2008/2009. He now works as a foundation year one doctor at Hull Royal Infirmary. His medical interests lie in the field of ophthalmology. Graham undertook a quality-improvement project at Hull Royal Infirmary in ophthalmology.

Dr Priha Shukla

Priha graduated from the University of Manchester's School of Medicine in July 2011 with an MB ChB. Her medical interests currently lie in the field of palliative care. She is currently working in The Christie Hospital in Manchester as a foundation year two doctor, having already developed an impressive reputation during foundation year one at the University Hospital of South Manchester.

Professor Peter McCollum

Peter is professor of vascular surgery at Hull York Medical School. He has extensive experience in examining at all levels of medical and surgical training and regularly examines overseas. He has examined medical student OSCEs at Hull York Medical School, University of Dundee, Nottingham University, Sheffield University and Leeds University. He is a member of council and deputy exam convenor in the Royal College of Surgeons of Edinburgh. He has published widely, and his principal research interest lies in clinical outcome.

Acknowledgements

Colleagues from many specialties throughout medicine and surgery have contributed to the production of this book. Each chapter has been written by well-respected doctors and reviewed by experts in their respective field. We would like to thank those who have helped us either in writing or reviewing chapters in this book:

Dr Thomas Hansen (foundation year one) and Mr Kevin Morris (consultant neurosurgeon) for helping to write and review the neurology chapter, respectively; Dr Rasmeet Kainth (foundation year one) and Dr Suparna Dasgupta (consultant paediatrician) for helping to write and review the paediatric chapter, respectively; Dr Amit Sindhi (specialist registrar psychiatrist) for helping to write and review the psychiatry chapter; Mr Sachchidananda Maiti and Mrs Wendy Noble (consultant obstetricians and gynaecologists) for helping to review the obstetrics and gynaecology chapter; Dr Rachel Gorodkin (consultant rheumatologist) for helping to review the musculoskeletal and general medicine chapters; Dr Patrick Newman (general practitioner) for helping to review the general medicine chapter; Dr David Ahearn (registrar general medicine) for reviewing the gastroenterology chapter; Professor Andrew Clark (professor of cardiology) and Dr Simon Hart (consultant respiratory physician) for helping to review the cardiorespiratory chapter; Mr Sigurd Kraus (consultant urologist) for helping to review the urology chapter; Mr Jim Innes (consultant ophthalmologist) for helping to review the ophthalmology chapter; and Dr Jordan Fletcher for his graphical expertise in creating the figure used in this book.

List of abbreviations

A&E	accident and emergency department
ABG	arterial blood gas
ACE	angiotensin-converting enzyme
ACS	acute coronary syndrome
ADHD	attention deficit hyperactivity disorder
ALP	alkaline phosphatase
ALS	advanced life support
ALT	alanine transaminase
ANA	anti-nuclear antibodies
ANCA	anti-neutrophil cytoplasmic antibodies
BMI	body mass index
BNP	brain natriuretic peptide
BPH	benign prostatic hyperplasia
BPPV	benign paroxysmal positional vertigo
CBT	cognitive behavioural therapy
CMV	cytomegalovirus
COCP	combined oral contraceptive pill
COPD	chronic obstructive pulmonary disorder
CRP	C-reactive protein
CT	computed tomography
CTD	connective tissue disorder
CTPA	computed tomography pulmonary angiography
CVS	cardiovascular system
DAT	dopamine transporter
DEXA	dual-energy X-ray absorptiometry
DH	drug history
DMARD	disease modifying anti-rheumatic drug
DVLA	driver and vehicle licensing agency
DVT	deep vein thrombosis
EBV	Epstein–Barr virus
ECG	electrocardiography
EEG	electroencephalography
eGFR	estimated glomerular filtration rate
ENT	ear, nose and throat
ESR	erythrocyte sedimentation rate
FAST	focused assessment with sonography for trauma

FBC	full blood count
FH	family history
FSH	follicle-stimulating hormone
G6PD	glucose-6-phosphate dehydrogenase
GIT	gastrointestinal tract
GORD	gastro-oesophageal reflux disease
GP	general practitioner
GT	glutamyl transferase
GTN	gliceryl trinitrate
GUM	genitourinary medicine
GUT	genitourinary tract
hCG	human chorionic gonadotropin
HDL	high-density lipoprotein
HIV	human immunodeficiency virus
HLA	human leucocyte antigen
HPC	history of presenting complaint
HPV	human papilloma virus
HRT	hormone replacement therapy
HSP	Henoch–Schönlein purpura
IBD	inflammatory bowel disease
IBS	irritable bowel syndrome
ICE	ideas, concerns and expectations
ICP	intracranial pressure
IHD	ischaemic heart disease
IM	intramuscular
IMB	intermenstrual bleeding
IV	intravenous
KUB	kidneys, ureter and bladder
LDL	low-density lipoprotein
LFT	liver function test
LH	luteinising hormone
LMN	lower motor neurone
LMP	last menstrual period
LOC	loss of consciousness
LRTI	lower respiratory tract infection
MDT	multidisciplinary team
MRI	magnetic resonance imaging
MS	musculoskeletal system
MSU	midstream urine sample
NAI	non-accidental injury
NS	nervous system
NSAID	non-steroidal anti-inflammatory drug
OSCE	objective structured clinical examination
OSLER	objective structured long examination record
PC	presenting complaint
PCB	post-coital bleeding

PCI	percutaneous coronary intervention
PCR	polymerase chain reaction
PE	pulmonary embolism
PET	positron emission tomography
PMB	post-menopausal bleeding
PMH	past medical history
PR	per rectal
PRN	pro re nata (as required)
PSA	prostate-specific antigen
PUO	pyrexia of unknown origin
PUVA	psoralen ultraviolet A (photochemotherapy)
PV	per vaginal
RA	rheumatoid arthritis
RS	respiratory system
SH	social history
SIADH	syndrome of inappropriate antidiuretic hormone hypersecretion
SLE	systemic lupus erythematosus
SP	simulated patient
SSRI	selective serotonin reuptake inhibitor
STI	sexually transmitted infection
TB	tuberculosis
TFT	thyroid function test
TNF	tumour necrosis factor
U&E	urea and electrolyte
UMN	upper motor neurone
URTI	upper respiratory tract infection
USS	ultrasound scan
UTI	urinary tract infection
VEGF	vascular endothelial growth factor
V/Q	ventilation/perfusion

Taking a focused history in OSCEs

An OSCE (objective, structured, clinical examination) is a tool that is increasingly used by undergraduate and postgraduate examining bodies to assess medical students and doctors at various stages of their careers. It is made up of a number of short encounters between the examinee and a scenario which may encompass a patient or be made up of a problem, such as an abnormal ECG. Many scenarios require the candidate to take a short history from a patient or, more often, simulated patient (SP) who is provided with an appropriate script and background to fulfil the role of patient. These stations are often referred to as 'information gathering' scenarios, but may also encompass 'information giving' scenarios. Indeed, some stations will combine both concepts, which may be separately assessed.

These OSCE encounters require the candidate to be extremely focused when taking the history; long-winded monologues from the patient will make the job of understanding the issues and later diagnosis very difficult, and the skill of a good candidate is to be found in the way they adapt the interview to gain the maximum information from the patient while at the same time adopting a listening and caring approach. Indeed, an OSCE history station is very much like a real-life situation for the average family physician, where they often have only 10 minutes to take a history, examine the patient and generate a working diagnosis with a management plan. As such, the Calgary–Cambridge model of interview is extremely valuable, but must be streamlined to allow the candidate time to make a differential diagnosis and formulate a working plan.

The key ingredients of the Calgary–Cambridge model are summarised below, as the model, or a variation thereof, is used and promoted in most medical schools throughout the UK. However, a more detailed description can be found elsewhere in most modern medical textbooks.

The Calgary–Cambridge model and the OSCE
Initiating the interview
- **Greeting:** greet patient and obtain patient's name
- **Introduction:** introduce self; describe your role and the reason for interview; obtain consent
- **Respect:** demonstrate interest, concern and respect for the patient as a person; ensure the patient's comfort
- **Non-verbal behaviour:** demonstrate an appropriate affect (e.g. eye contact,

posture and position, movement, facial expression, use of voice); in summary, 'be human'!

♦ **The opening question:** identify the patient's problem(s) or the issue(s) that the patient wishes to discuss (e.g. 'What concerns brought you to the hospital/ clinic' or 'What are the problems that you would like to discuss?') Find out what *their* main problem is (this might not be why they were referred to a clinic)

♦ **Listen to the patient's opening statement:** listen without interrupting or directing patient's response initially, although you may need to truncate this diplomatically in the OSCE!

♦ **Facilitative response:** encourage the patient's responses both verbally and non-verbally

♦ **Cues:** pick up verbal and non-verbal cues (body language, speech, facial expression, affect); look for props (medications, cigarette packets, internet printout, etc.)

♦ **Screening:** check and confirm the list of problems or issues that the patient wishes to cover ('What other problems have you noticed?' or 'Is there anything else you would like to bring to my attention?')

♦ **Agenda setting:** negotiate an agenda and a format of interview, taking both the patient's and physician's needs into account; in most OSCEs, this will be self-evident to both parties

Exploration of the patient's problems

♦ **Patient's narrative:** encourage the patient to tell their story from the beginning, within reason; clearly, if the patient is excessively verbose, they will need to be 'moved on' politely but firmly

♦ **Question style:** use both open-ended and closed questions; move appropriately from open to closed; this will be critical to getting through the agenda in an OSCE station, and you will probably find that most questions will need to be closed or semi-closed towards the end of the interview

♦ **Listening:** listen attentively; allow the patient to complete statements without interruption; leave space for the patient to think before answering or go on after pausing; this is sometimes an idealistic aspiration, however, and must be balanced against the need to 'deliver' in the OSCE station

♦ **Facilitative response:** facilitate the patient's responses verbally and non-verbally (use encouragement, silence, repetition, paraphrasing, interpretation)

♦ **Cues:** pick up verbal and non-verbal cues (body language, speech, facial expression, affect); check them out and acknowledge as appropriate (e.g. 'You seem tired')

♦ **Clarification:** clarify any statements which are vague (e.g. 'What do you mean by diarrhoea?')

♦ **Time framing:** establish the sequence of events clearly

♦ **Internal summary:** periodically recap to validate what the patient has said; allow the patient an opportunity to correct your interpretation and provide further information

◆ **Appropriate use of language:** use concise, clear and easily understood questions; avoid jargon

Exploration of the disease framework
◆ **Focused closed questions:** ask appropriate closed questions to explore facets of the history that have not emerged from the patient's story
◆ **Symptom analysis:** (e.g. pain) onset, site, radiation, character, severity, duration, frequency and periodicity, special times of occurrence, aggravating factors, relieving factors, associated features
◆ **Relevant systems enquiry:** ask questions relevant to the appropriate system being explored as well as a quick check on other systems (systems review)

Exploration of the patient's perspective
◆ **Ideas and concerns:** assess the patient's ideas (i.e. beliefs re causality) and concerns regarding each problem; establish their *main* concern
◆ **Effects:** determine the effects of the problem(s) on the patient's activities of daily living and psyche
◆ **Expectations:** establish what the patient expects from the consultation
◆ **Feelings and thoughts:** encourage the expression of the patient's feelings and thoughts, but do not just ask 'What are your thoughts?' as this can often appear crass and rather mechanical

Explanation and planning (often comes under the heading of 'information giving' in an OSCE format)
◆ **Provide the correct amount and type of information:** adjust for the ability of the patient to understand/assimilate information; even the brightest of patients only remembers so much
◆ **Assess the patient's starting point:** establish the patient's current understanding of their problem (if any) at the outset; establish how much the patient wants to know
◆ **Chunks and checks:** give information in digestible chunks; check for understanding; use the patient's response as a guide to how much more is required
◆ **Give any explanation at appropriate times:** try to provide examples and signposts to help patient remember explanations
◆ **Use explicit categorisation or signposting of information chunks:** e.g. 'There are three important things that I would like to tell you about' (try to make the most important issue the first one)
◆ **Check the patient's understanding:** e.g. by asking patient to restate in their own words; clarify if necessary
◆ **Use repetition and summarise:** to reinforce and embed information in patients
◆ **Use visual aids:** diagrams, models, written information and instructions
◆ **Use simple language:** use concise, easily understood statements; avoid jargon

Achieving a shared understanding: incorporating the patient's illness framework

+ **Relate explanations to the patient's illness framework:** to previously expressed concerns and expectations
+ **Provide opportunities and encourage the patient to contribute:** by asking questions, seeking clarification or expressing doubts; respond appropriately
+ **Use verbal and non-verbal cues:** e.g. the patient's feedback; ask questions; beware information overload and subsequent distress
+ **Elicit and assess the patient's reactions and feelings:** re information given, terms used; acknowledge and clarify where necessary

Planning: shared decision making

+ **Share own thoughts:** ideas, thought processes and dilemmas
+ **Involve the patient:** make suggestions rather than directives; 'What would you like?'
+ **Encourage the patient:** to contribute their thoughts, ideas, suggestions and preferences
+ **Negotiate:** negotiate a mutually acceptable plan
+ **Offer choice:** where desired, ask the patient to make informed choices and decisions
+ **Check with the patient:** if concerns have been addressed

Closure

+ **End summary:** summarises session briefly and clarifies plan of care
+ **Contract:** agrees with patient re next steps for patient and physician
+ **Safety net:** explains possible unexpected outcomes, alternatives, when and how to seek help
+ **Final check:** check that patient agrees and is comfortable with plan and asks if any corrections, questions or other items to discuss

The above is of course a council of perfection! Clearly, there is often a gap between what is desirable and what is feasible to deliver in the OSCE exam setting with regard to history taking. The successful candidate is one who can combine the ethos of the Calgary–Cambridge methodology with a structured and functional approach such that key elements of the history are not left out. A useful synopsis of such an approach is shown on pp. 5–6.

It is important to remember that patients are inherently unreliable (as indeed are medical students and doctors), and so internal cross-checking of event dates, past medical problems, etc. is a very useful discipline. A simple example of this is hypertension, which will not be admitted by many patients simply because they consider that they no longer have it as they are now on antihypertensive medication. Use medications as a way of cross-checking the patient's past medical history. Thus, L-thyroxine in the list of medications would indicate that the patient has hypothyroidism, even if not originally volunteered.

There is an understandable danger of becoming too mechanical while information gathering. Students need to do more than just 'go through the motions' during the OSCE. A flat affect with little empathy comes across clearly to examiners and will not help the cause. Although it can be difficult to reconcile some scenarios with a clinical problem (e.g. a clearly normal SP giving a history of jaundice), every effort should be made to consider the scenario in a real-life context.

In each of the following chapters, there will be a brief description of the problem and an outline of the key factors in the approach to the history needed for that particular problem. There is inevitably some repetition, as certain elements such as initiating the interview (introduction, cues, screening, agenda setting, etc.) are common to all scenarios.

An active problem list to identify core issues that need to be addressed and remembered is very valuable. Some will be background issues (like hypertension) and not seen by the patient as a problem, while others may be very important from the patient's perspective (e.g. nausea, leg pain). Remember also that patients may well have more than one cause for their symptom. For example, leg pain may be due to a patient's arthritis and/or atherosclerosis. A careful history will identify two distinct types of pain and allow this to be identified and clarified.

In the information giving/explanation and planning sections, it is vital to remember that most patients attend a doctor for reassurance. Thus, this should underscore the dialogue where at all possible.

For the purposes of this book, examination has intentionally been left out, as this is well covered in other textbooks. Clearly, in many OSCE scenarios, history and examination go alongside one another. However, it remains the case that a well-taken history will guide the candidate to a focused and relevant examination; indeed, in many cases, a well-taken history alone can provide the diagnosis without any examination.

In some stations, the emphasis will also be on information giving. It is important here to provide patient reassurance and information if this is asked of you. Finally, you should try to effect a proper closure to the interview, even when in an OSCE. Consider using phrases such as: 'Is there anything that you didn't understand?' or 'Are there any questions you would like me to answer?' to round off your history.

The structure of these scenarios can easily be used to develop an appropriate approach to the OSLER, which is used in some medical schools alongside the OSCE, either for formative or summative assessment.

A framework for a structured history and examination
Patient's problems
List current active medical and other problems.

Medical	*Patient's perspective (ICE)*
Complaint events and time scales	Ideas & beliefs
Symptoms	Concerns
Specific system review	Expectations
	Effects on life/activities
	Feelings

Past medical history (including injuries)

Drug history

Allergies

Family history

Social history (smoking, drinking, recreational drugs, weight)

Personal (marital status, children, support, housing, work)

Systems review
- GIT
- GUT
- RS
- CVS
- NS
- MS
- Skin

Physical examination

Differential diagnosis
- Working diagnosis
- Certainty/uncertainty

Management plan
- Natural history of problem
- Treatment possibilities
- Investigations
- Time scales

Patient discussion/contract
- Explanation & clarification
- Reassurance
- Closure

General OSCE tips

Tips from recently qualified doctors

1. **Practise past stations with a small group of friends**
   - Two to three friends is ideal – one student, one patient and possibly one examiner to note what you have and haven't done well
   - Come up with a list of past stations and potential other stations and test your friends in a pressurised environment to simulate the real thing
   - Watch your friends closely – you will pick up things from others that you wouldn't have thought of yourself

2. **Practical revision**
   - Go on the wards to see patients with stomas, fistulas, etc. before your exams – if you haven't seen something before, it is usually obvious to the examiner
   - Revising from books and notes should only supplement your practical revision for OSCEs

3. **Use your reading time before each station efficiently**
   - Compose yourself and do not dwell on past stations – the great thing about OSCEs is you have a chance to start afresh with a different examiner every station
   - In your reading time, think carefully about what the question is asking you to do – examiners will get annoyed if you do not follow the instructions carefully
     - Is it a focused history, examination with a few pertinent questions, examination with no questions allowed or other?
     - If it is an examination, have they asked you only to examine one aspect or a complete examination? If in doubt about the instructions, ask the examiner
   - In your reading time, ask yourself what things you often forget when practising this type of station so you can remember in the real thing
   - In spotter stations (i.e. stations where you are presented with patients who often exhibit pathognomonic signs), your instructions may read along the lines of 'Please examine this patient's hand/knee/lower limb, etc. and give your diagnosis . . .' Use your reading time to come up with potential diagnoses you might see when you walk in, to prevent yourself drawing a blank as you walk in

4. **Wash your hands before and after seeing each patient/simulated patient!**
   + Practise doing this before each station, and make sure you point out to your friends when they have failed to do so – hand hygiene is very important, and students may be marked down for a failure to comply with this

5. **Be friendly to your examiners**
   + Smile and make eye contact with your examiners
   + They are more likely to be communicative with you if you are communicative with them

6. **Be friendly to your patients**
   + Take time to introduce yourself to the patient and establish some rapport (if they like you, they may even end up helping you along the way)
   + I would introduce myself and then give the patient an 'icebreaker' – e.g. 'If you have any questions at any point, feel free to ask, and I'll happily go through them with you. Otherwise, you can feel free to ignore me completely if you wish!' This would often draw a laugh from the patient (and sometimes also the examiner) and help establish a relationship with the patient
   + When allowed to ask questions, be sure to ask how their condition has affected their activities of daily living

7. **Don't panic in tricky stations**
   + Remember, if you find a station hard, don't panic; the chances are everyone else will find it hard too. Think of these stations as opportunities to gain extra marks, as many students will freeze in these stations

Tips from experienced examiners

1. **Forget about your previous station**
   + Remember, each station is completely separate
   + No one knows how well you did in the past station (including you and your next examiner), so put it out of your mind and focus on the next station
   + The only way the examiner may think you have generally performed poorly is by your demeanour if you let a 'bad' station affect you

2. **Professionalism is important**
   + Treat each patient/simulated patient with respect and use eye contact
   + Do not just spend time looking at paper/results – if there is a patient/ simulated patient in there, you are expected to act professionally, as you would in reality

3. **Look around for clues in each station**
   + Disease identifiers, e.g. walking aids, inhalers, oxygen, cardiac monitors, insulin pumps
   + Are there any props lying around – if so, use them, as it is likely to be on the examiner's marking criteria

4. **If in doubt about what is expected of you, seek clarification**
   + Examiners want you to pass and will usually try to point you in the right direction

- The worst that can happen is they will say, 'Do as you see fit!'
- An example for when you might seek clarification – you are told to examine the 'chest' (usually synonymous with a respiratory examination), but see a sternotomy scar. Point out that you see the sternotomy scar, which would most likely indicate coronary artery bypass grafting or a valve replacement, and ask if they would like you to conduct a cardiovascular examination or a respiratory examination

5. **Talk to your examiner unless instructed not to do so**
   - Most examiners like students to talk through what they are doing as they go along
   - It helps to signpost things for the examiner that are paramount to the station
   - Some examiners may ask you not to talk as you go along and prefer you simply to present at the end. If this happens, do not be put off by it

Tips for approaching a history-taking OSCE station

The start
1. **Have a system** – if facing an unfamiliar station, consider adopting a basic framework such as SOCRATES; this will show the examiner you are thinking systematically
2. **Good communication skills** – even in what may feel like a contrived or unreal situation, it is important to show the patient that you are listening empathetically to their problems and concerns
3. **ABCDE approach** – start your ABCDE approach if the patient appears critically unwell (e.g. haematemesis)

The middle
1. **History of presenting complaint** – this is the most important part of most histories, and you should aim to spend half of the allocated time on it
2. **Summarise when stuck** – not only can this buy you some time to think of your next move, it comforts the patient and examiner by letting them know you have been listening and may also elucidate any area that was unclear
3. **Respond to cues** – do not ignore cues. You have your agenda, but so does the patient. SPs will often try to point you in the right direction if you let them. Let them air their concerns as they arise; do not ignore them. Acknowledge and legitimise them, answer them to the best of your ability and come back to them later in the history to see if their concerns have changed at all
4. **Ideas, concerns and expectations** – you will be expected to ask about the patient's perspective on their illness; in the modern consultation, it is important that you listen to the patient's concerns attentively – this may even help prompt you down a line of questioning
5. **Review of systems** – can be helpful if after the history of presenting complaint you are still very unclear as to possible diagnoses; it may help you realise that you have been barking up the wrong tree entirely and help you shift the focus of the history before it is too late!

The end

1. **To finish** – at the end of every history, summarise, ask the patient if you have missed anything or if they have any questions or concerns you haven't already answered
2. **Differential diagnosis** – top marks for a history often come at the end with how you present your diagnosis and differentials; comment on working diagnosis and what parts of the history made you think that and not others
3. **Investigations and managements** – the investigations and management listed in this book are designed to cover the most likely differentials; they are not necessarily comprehensive, nor do they all need to be utilised in every case (in an exam, you should only say the ones relevant to the scenario you are presented with if/when asked by the examiner)

General medicine

Pain 14
Tiredness 16
Fever 20
Rash 24
Bruising 28

Pain

HPC

O'SOCRATES

- **Open question** – Can you tell me a bit more about your pain?
- **Site** – Where exactly do you get this pain? Can you point to it precisely?
- **Onset** – When did this pain start? Did it come on suddenly or gradually?
- **Character** – What does the pain feel like?
- **Radiation** – Does the pain go anywhere else?
- **Associated features** (depending on type of pain) – this could include a systems review
- **Timing** – Is the pain there all the time or does it come and go? Is there any particular time where you have noticed you get the pain? Have you ever had this pain before?
- **Exacerbating/relieving factors** – What brings the pain on? Does anything make it worse? Does anything make it better? Have you taken anything to relieve the pain?
- **Severity** – If you had to rate the pain now from 1 to 10, with 10 being the worst pain you can imagine, how would you score the pain? How would you score it at its worst? How have your symptoms affected your day-to-day life?

PMH

- Do you suffer from any medical conditions?

DH

- Are you currently taking any medications?
- Do you have any allergies?

FH

- Do any conditions run in the family?
- Has anyone else in your family suffered from this kind of pain? Were they diagnosed?

SH

- Do you drink alcohol? How much do you drink in a week?
- Do you smoke? How many cigarettes do you smoke a day? For how long have you smoked?
- Are you currently employed? *If so*, what do you do for a living?
- What is your current situation at home? How are you coping at home?

An alternative method

There are several ways of approaching any history. Here we have shown the SOCRATES mnemonic for taking the history (whilst emphasising the importance of starting with an open question). We show this method as it is a very useful way of structuring a history, and providing you don't miss out any steps, you should not miss out anything important in the history of the presenting complaint. It is, however, not the only way you can structure the history.

Some physicians find it more useful to take a chronological approach, where they start from the beginning of when the patient first experienced the pain and chronologically advance to see how it has progressed. Other physicians have different methods.

In practice, the two approaches are effectively amalgamated into an order that flows more easily than the order in SOCRATES. An alternative approach is shown below.

1. Ask open questions about the pain to elicit as much information as possible before direct closed questioning (they will almost always immediately tell you the *site* of the pain and often the *character* as well as gauging an idea of *severity*)
2. Ascertain a chronological order of events in your head to help understand what is going on
    a. When did the pain start? *Onset*
    b. Has it always been there since it started or has it come and gone? When do you notice the pain? *Timing*
    c. How has the pain progressed since you first noticed it? *Severity*
3. Ascertain a detailed description of the pain
    a. What does the pain feel like? *Character*
    b. Does it go anywhere else? *Radiation*
    c. Can you think of anything that brings the pain on? Does anything make it worse? Does anything make it better? *Exacerbating/relieving factors*
4. Finally, ask about *Associated features*
    a. Have you noticed any other symptoms?
    b. Ask specific questions related to both the systems involved and a review of other systems (a few short questions for each system)
    c. Ascertain a timeline for these symptoms as well

Tiredness
HPC
O'SOCRATES

+ **Open question** – Can you tell me more about what's been going on? What exactly do you mean when you say you feel tired/fatigued?
+ **Specific reason** – Can you think of any reason for feeling tired?
+ **Onset** – When did you first notice this? How were you before then?
+ **Character of sleep** – How are you sleeping?
+ **Refreshment** – Does sleep refresh you?
+ **Associated features** – *See screening questions later*
+ **Timing** – Do you ever not feel tired? If so, when?
+ **Exacerbating/relieving factors** – Does anything worsen your tiredness? (e.g. exercise, emotional stress)
+ **Severity** – How has this affected you?

ICE
What do you think is causing your tiredness? Are you particularly concerned about anything? What is your biggest concern you'd like dealt with?

Screening questions
+ Aside from your tiredness, how have you been feeling? Have you had any other symptoms? Have you been feeling feverish or generally unwell? If so, in what way?
+ **Viral illness** – Have you had a sore throat or a cold recently?
+ **Cancer** – Have you noticed a cough? Change in bowel habit? Any lumps? Problems urinating? Have you noticed any change in your weight over the past few months? If so, was this intentional or not? How is your appetite?
+ **Hypothyroidism** – Do you find yourself feeling cold even when others say it is warm?
+ **Diabetes** – Have you had to go to the toilet more often recently? Do you find yourself feeling constantly thirsty despite drinking more than you used to?
+ **Depression** – Have you been suffering from low mood recently? If so, for how long? Do you have any hobbies you enjoy doing?
+ **Chronic fatigue syndrome/fibromyalgia** – Do you have any pain in your muscles? Headaches? How is your memory and concentration?
+ **Menorrhagia (anaemia)** – Do you suffer from heavy periods?
+ *Ask follow-up questions as appropriate where a positive response is given.*

PMH
+ Do you suffer from any medical or psychiatric conditions?
+ *Ask specifically about diabetes, thyroid disease, IBS, fibromyalgia and any past history of cancer*

DH

+ Are you taking any medications? Have any of these been changed recently?
+ Are you taking any over-the-counter medications?
+ Do you have any allergies?

FH

+ Do any conditions run in your family?
+ *Ask specifically about diabetes, thyroid disease and cancer*

SH

+ Are you currently working? If so, what do you do?
+ Do you smoke? Drink? Take recreational drugs?
+ Who is at home with you?

Important points

+ Be empathetic to the patient's concerns and how the symptoms have affected them. Communication skills are vital in histories like this one
+ In this history the cause will often be a non-sinister one; however, you are unlikely to be awarded top marks unless you have been seen to be actively ruling out other causes

Differential diagnosis

Environmental – the most common cause

+ Poor sleeping environment or an unstructured sleeping routine
+ Working long hours with stressful jobs ('burnout')
+ Having small children and/or being a carer for someone

Viral illness (non-specific)

+ Short history of flu-like symptoms that if left a week will disappear by themselves
+ More severe cases can result in a prolonged postviral state of fatigue (*see also* chronic fatigue syndrome, p. 18)

Infectious mononucleosis

+ The 'kissing disease' is caused by Epstein–Barr virus – suspect in adolescents
+ History of sore throat and flu-like symptoms that persist longer than would be expected from other common viruses

Anaemia

+ Blood loss is the most common cause of a microcytic anaemia – remember to consider NSAIDs, menorrhagia and colorectal carcinoma as likely underlying causes
+ Chronic disease can cause a normocytic picture (anaemia of chronic disease)
+ Folate/B_{12} deficiency, hypothyroidism and alcoholism can cause a macrocytic picture

Hypothyroidism

◆ Weight gain despite decreased appetite, intolerance of cold, constipation, menstrual irregularities, low mood and feeling slow are among many features
◆ There may be a family history of thyroid disease or just autoimmune disease
◆ Usually female and middle-aged

Diabetes mellitus

◆ Polyuria, polydipsia, increased appetite and weight loss
◆ Presentation with tiredness is most commonly seen in type 1 – usually a young adolescent presenting for the first time, but can also be a known type 1 diabetic who is not taking their insulin
◆ Type 2 can also present with fatigue, but is much more likely than type 1 to be asymptomatic

Cancer

◆ Constitutional symptoms such as weight loss, decreased appetite and fever
◆ The big four causes of cancer are breast, prostate, lung and colorectal carcinomas
◆ Suspect in patients with significant weight loss, symptoms and risk factors for a particular cancer (e.g. suspect lung cancer in a patient with haemoptysis and breathlessness who has smoked for 40 years)

Cardiac, renal or liver failure

◆ Ankle oedema and symptoms specific to the failing system
◆ Past history of cardiac, renal or liver disease is likely to be present

Depression

◆ Core symptoms: low mood, anhedonia and fatigue present for > 2 weeks
◆ Typical symptoms: sleep disturbance, early morning waking (> 2 hours earlier than usual), decreased appetite and weight loss (> 10%)

Chronic fatigue syndrome

◆ Persistent fatigue for more than 6 months in a previously healthy individual that is not due to ongoing physical exertion, not relieved by rest and cannot be explained by another medical condition
◆ Myalgia, headaches, sore throat and poor concentration and memory
◆ There may be a past history of irritable bowel syndrome and/or fibromyalgia
◆ Bear in mind that fatigue is also a prominent symptom of fibromyalgia, although usually less dominant than the symptoms of musculoskeletal pain

Iatrogenic

◆ Many medications can cause fatigue (particularly beta blockers) – ask if any medications have been changed recently

Investigations

- Cardiorespiratory examination and breast/PR examination (if breast/colorectal cancer suspected)
- Check for a palpable thyroid
- FBC, U&Es, LFTs, TFTs, blood glucose, ESR and CRP
- Urinalysis for diabetes and renal failure
- Monospot test for infectious mononucleosis
- Serum ferritin/B_{12}/folate if evidence of anaemia
- Upper and/or lower GIT investigations if unexplained iron-deficiency anaemia
- Based on clinical suspicion – mammography/USS and biopsy for breast cancer; PSA for prostatic cancer; chest X-ray and bronchoscopy for lung cancer; faecal occult blood and colonoscopy for colorectal cancer

Management

- Personal circumstances – sleep hygiene (a structured sleeping routine); can work situation be altered? Would counselling be beneficial?
- Virus/infectious mononucleosis – bed rest and hydration
- Anaemia – treat depending on cause
- Hypothyroidism – thyroxine
- Diabetes mellitus type 1 – insulin therapy (consider insulin pump if poorly controlled); type 2 – appropriate diabetic medication and/or insulin
- Cancer – refer onwards for specialist management
- Cardiac, renal or liver failure – treat depending on cause
- Depression – SSRIs and CBT
- Chronic fatigue syndrome – non-vigorous exercise (excessive exercise will exacerbate the condition) and CBT

Fever

HPC

Clarify HOT

- **Clarify** – What exactly do you mean when you say you feel feverish? Can you describe exactly how you feel?
  - Do you feel hot or cold? Have you been shivering? Night sweats?
- **How** are you feeling generally? Any nausea? Pain anywhere?
- **Onset** – How long have you felt like this?
- **Timing/triggers** – Does the fever come and go or is it constant? Does anything bring it on?

ICE

- Have you got any idea what might be causing the fever? Is there anything you are particularly worried about?

Infection

Note: These are screening questions; if a positive answer is given to any of them, this necessitates further questioning about the symptom in question.

- **URTI/LRTI** – Do you have a cough or shortness of breath? Any sputum?
- **UTI** – Do you have any pain on urination? Are you going more frequently?
- **Meningitis** – Do you have a headache? Neck stiffness? A rash?
- **Gastrointestinal cause** – Have you had any diarrhoea or vomiting?
- **STI** – Have you recently had unprotected sex with a new partner?
- **Tropical** – Have you travelled anywhere abroad recently? Any insect bites?

Malignancy

- **Constitutional** – Have you lost any weight recently? How is your appetite?
- **Haematological** – Have you been bruising or bleeding more easily? Have you been getting lots of infections?
- **Bowel** – Have you had any change in bowel habit?
- **Lung** – Have you had a cough? Have you brought up any blood?
- **Breast** – Have you noticed any lumps or changes in your breasts?
- **Prostate/bladder/kidney** – Have you passed any blood in your urine?

Autoimmune/other conditions

- **Inflammatory arthritis** – Are any of your joints or muscles stiff or painful?
- **Temporal arteritis** – Is it painful when you chew food?
- **Vasculitis** – Have you noticed any skin lesions? Any ulcers or changes in the colour of your fingers/toes?
- **CTD** – Do your hands change colour in the cold? Do you suffer with dry eyes or a dry mouth?
- **DVT** – Have either of your legs become swollen, painful and hot?

PMH
♦ Do you have any medical conditions?
♦ *Ask specifically about arthritis, HIV, previous cancer and recent surgery*

DH
♦ Are you taking any medications?
♦ Have any of these been changed recently?
♦ Do you have any allergies?

FH
♦ Do any conditions run in the family?
♦ *Ask specifically about autoimmune disease, diabetes, cancer and thyroid disease*
♦ Do any friends or family have infections at the moment?

SH
♦ What is your occupation?
♦ Do you smoke (have you ever smoked)? How many do you smoke a day? For how long have you smoked?
♦ Do you drink alcohol? How much do you drink in a week?

Important points
♦ This would be a tricky station to face in an OSCE, as fever is a non-specific symptom; the initial approach should be to outline its history and then to systematically search for a cause, making it clear you are ruling out sinister causes such as malignancy and serious infections (e.g. meningitis)
♦ Start by asking one or two open questions so you can get as much information from them as possible, but direct questioning with closed questions will then be important, particularly in the time-pressurised scenario of an OSCE
♦ It is important in such a station that you make it clear to the examiner that you are systematically ruling out many different causes – even if you do not get the diagnosis, this may be sufficient to impress and gain very good marks

Differential diagnosis
Fever is normally due to a self-limiting viral infection or uncomplicated bacterial infection. However, where no cause can be found after sufficient time and investigations, pyrexia of unknown origin exists. The causes of this can come under the headings of infection, malignancy or autoimmune, as outlined below.

Infections
Tuberculosis (TB)
♦ Weight loss, night sweats, lymphadenopathy and haemoptysis
♦ Previous TB exposure, chronic alcoholism, homeless patients, intravenous (IV) drug abusers and a compromised immune system are risk factors

Infectious endocarditis
+ Non-specific malaise and flu-like illness, as well as cardiac and embolic symptoms such as shortness of breath or systemic infarctions
+ Classically, patients may have recently been to the dentist where inoculation takes place and/or have pre-existing valvular disease

Malignancy
+ Weight loss and cachexia, as well as other red flags, such as melaena, haemoptysis and haematuria are likely to be present for specific cancers
+ Haematological cancers often present with fever, as well as bruising, recurrent infections and anaemia

Autoimmune
Temporal arteritis/polymyalgia rheumatica
+ Throbbing headache and tenderness over the temple/bilateral stiffness or pain in the shoulders, pelvic girdle and neck
+ In both cases, the patient is almost always over 65 years old

Rheumatoid arthritis
+ Symmetrical polyarthritis, typically affecting small joints
+ Most commonly seen in females
+ Hot, swollen and tender joints with morning stiffness

Connective tissue disease (e.g. SLE)
+ Sicca symptoms (e.g. Raynaud's, dry eyes and dry mouth) and fatigue are prominent features
+ Arthralgia, rashes, renal and lung involvement are common among CTDs, although any organ can be affected

Vasculitis
+ Skin lesions (possibly necrotic), urticaria, oedema, arthralgia and other systemic features may be present

Miscellaneous
Drug-induced fever
+ Some patients have a hypersensitivity to drugs which results in a fever alone rather than anaphylaxis
+ Consider this in any patient with no other localising signs or symptoms who developed fever after starting/increasing the dose of a medication

Familial Mediterranean fever
+ An inherited condition, autosomal recessive, more common in Mediterranean ethnicities, particularly subsets of Jewish communities
+ Causes recurrent bouts of fever, abdominal pain and pleuritic chest pain, as well as numerous other inflammatory reactions, e.g. joint pains

Investigations

- Bloods – FBC, U&Es, LFTs, TFTs, ESR, CRP and serum ferritin
- Autoimmune screen, including rheumatoid factor, ANA and ANCA
- Blood cultures
- Urinalysis – urine microscopy, culture and sensitivity
- Chest X-ray
- Mantoux test and QuantiFERON-TB Gold for TB
- CT, MRI or USS depending on suspected malignancy or abscess
- Temporal artery biopsy
- Colonoscopy and upper GIT endoscopy
- Echocardiography
- Doppler

Management

- Tuberculosis is treated using 6 months of isoniazid and rifampicin, with the addition for the first 2 months of pyrazinamide and ethambutol
- Infectious endocarditis – IV gentamicin plus another IV antibiotic (depending on the results of blood cultures and suspected organism)
- Malignancy – surgery, chemotherapy, radiotherapy and/or palliation
- Rheumatoid arthritis – methotrexate first-line, with sulphasalazine and leflunomide as second-line therapies; anti-TNF drugs if these fail
- Temporal arteritis and polymyalgia rheumatica – high-dose oral steroids
- SLE and vasculitis – immunosuppressive therapy

Rash

HPC

O'SOCRATES

- **Open question** – Can you describe the rash for me?
- **Site** – Where is the rash?
- **Onset** – When did it start? How did it start?
- **Colour** – What colour is it? Does it look red and angry?
- **Radiation** – Does it spread anywhere else or is it just in the one area?
- **Associated features** – Is it itchy? Is it sore or painful? Any discharge? Any burning or numbness? Does the rash disappear or go white if you press it?
- **Timing** – Is it always there? Has it changed over time? Have you had a similar rash before?
- **Exacerbating/relieving factors** – Can you think of anything that triggers it? Are you using any new hand creams, perfumes, washing powders or other substances likely to contact the skin? Does anything make it better or worse? Is it worse when you are in the sun?
- **Severity** – How is it affecting your day-to-day life?

Systemic symptoms
Note: These are screening questions; if a positive answer is given to any of them, this necessitates further questioning about the symptom in question.
- **Constitutional** – Have you been feeling unwell recently? Have you been feverish? Any lethargy, loss of appetite or nausea?
- **URTI/LRTI** – Any recent infections? Recent cough with phlegm?
- **UTI** – Any problems passing water?
- **Meningitis** – Any headache? Neck stiffness?
- **Autoimmune** – Do you suffer from pain in your joints or your back? Painfully cold hands? Dry eyes or mouth? Ulcers? Hair loss?

ICE
- Have you got any idea what might be causing the rash? Is there anything you are particularly worried about? What is the main concern you would like dealt with?

PMH
- Do you suffer from any medical conditions?
- *Ask specifically about eczema, lupus, psoriasis, arthritis and bleeding disorders*
- Any previous dermatological history, diagnoses or investigations?

DH
- Are you currently taking any medications? Any herbal medicines or over-the-counter medicines?
- Have there been any changes to your medications in the last few months?
- Do you have any allergies?

FH

+ Does anyone else in the family suffer with a similar condition?
+ Do any conditions run in the family?
+ *Ask specifically about rashes, allergies, arthritis (if so, clarify which arthritis)*

SH

+ What do you do for a job? Do you come into contact with any harmful or irritating materials? Do you wear protection?
+ Does anyone else in the house, or any other close contacts, have the same rash?
+ What is your home situation like? Is it crowded? Is it clean?
+ Do you smoke? Do you drink alcohol?

Important points

+ Firstly, try to gain as much information as possible from the patient using open questions and gain a thorough description from the patient before firing closed questions
+ Some patients may walk in with visual clues (even simulated patients!), e.g. they may be wearing a hat to conceal their scalp psoriasis. If something appears different, then comment on it and ask the patient about it – this will gain the interest of your examiner
+ Dermatological disorders can have a profound effect on the patient's psychological health, particularly in young females – be sure to ask how it is affecting them and about their concerns
+ Although examination of the rash is crucial, this should not be at the expense of a good history

Differential diagnosis

Psoriasis

+ Typically, well-demarcated red scaly plaques (chronic plaque psoriasis), but pustular, guttate, erythrodermic and nail psoriatic varieties also exist
+ Usually found on extensor surfaces
+ Family history often present
+ May be itchy; there may be an associated arthropathy and nail changes

Atopic eczema

+ Suggested by a red exudative or scaly lesion, often with vesicles
+ Usually on the flexor surfaces, face and neck, favouring skin creases
+ Often very itchy – there may be evidence of excoriation or lichenification
+ Family history of atopy such as asthma, hay fever or drug allergies

Contact dermatitis

+ Similar in presentation to eczema, but with an irritant or allergic aetiology
+ Commonly found on hands and may be linked to occupation, e.g. a cleaner who reacts to soapy water

Seborrhoeic dermatitis
- A scaly, greasy, itchy rash that typically affects the scalp and face. Areas of the face affected include the nasolabial folds, eyebrows and eyelids
- Dandruff is a common finding
- Can occur in newborns, where it is known as cradle cap

Viral-induced rash
- The most common cause of a maculopapular rash in children
- Usually a history of a preceding viral illness or malaise
- The rash blanches when pressed, and is not itchy or sore

Varicella zoster
- Diffuse, itchy and painful vesicular and pustular lesions at different stages of development
- Shingles presents in immunocompromised adults in a dermatomal distribution
- Herpes zoster ophthalmicus may occur in trigeminal nerve involvement

Purpuric rash
- Small purple raised spots on the skin that do not blanch when pressed
- Wide range of causes, including meningococcal septicaemia
- Henoch–Schönlein purpura affects lower extremities and buttocks of children

Urticaria
- White, itchy papule surrounded by erythema – multiple, localised or diffuse
- They occur very acutely, usually as a reaction to a topical allergen
- Can progress to anaphylaxis, which may result in angioedema
- Patients may have a history of hypersensitivity

Cellulitis
- Well-demarcated erythematous rash, with swelling, warmth and tenderness
- Usually localised, often on the legs. There may be tracking, whereby the rash spreads along the routes of the lymphatics
- Fever, tachycardia and malaise may be present

Investigations
- Full dermatological examination
- Dermoscopy for detailed examination of lesion
- Diascopy to reveal non-blanching rashes
- Biopsy to confirm diagnosis
- Skin scrapings for fungal infections
- Skin-prick and patch testing
- Swabs if infection is suspected
- Wood's light can help highlight certain fungal infections, such as tinea capitus
- Autoantibody screen
- FBC and clotting screen to rule out bleeding disorders

Management

♦ A purpuric rash is managed based on its cause, e.g. antibiotics for meningococcal septicaemia or splenectomy for treatment of recurrent idiopathic thrombocytopaenic purpura

♦ Seborrhoeic dermatitis – topical steroid cream for flare-ups, and antifungal shampoo or cream for regular use to reduce relapses

♦ Psoriasis – avoid excess drying of skin; encourage sun exposure; topical steroid and vitamin D analogue preparations; ultraviolet light/PUVA therapy; coal tar; methotrexate and cyclosporin are extreme options

♦ Dermatitis – avoid precipitants, including soaps, creams and perfumes; topical moisturisers; topical steroids for flare-ups

♦ Herpes zoster – acyclovir within 72 hours' onset of rash

♦ Cellulitis – oral antibiotics, e.g. flucloxacillin for *Staphylococcus aureus*

Bruising

HPC

O'SOCRATES

+ **Open question** – Can you tell me what has been going on?
+ **Site** – Where are the bruises? How many are there?
+ **Onset** – When did you first notice the bruising? How has it progressed?
+ **Character** – Can you describe the bruises? Are they large or like pinpricks?
+ **Radiation** – Do you have any bruises elsewhere?
+ **Associated features** – *see later*
+ **Timing** – Have you suffered from easy bruising before?
+ **Exacerbating/relieving factors** – Any recent bumps or injuries?
+ **Severity** – Have you been feeling particularly ill and tired recently?

Bleeding history

+ Do you tend to bleed very easily and for long periods of time when cut?
+ Are your periods very heavy? Did you bleed much after giving birth?
+ Have you ever had any trouble with massive bleeding after an operation?
+ Do you get lots of nosebleeds?
+ Is there ever any blood in your stools? Any blood in your urine?
+ Have you ever suffered with bleeding into the joints or muscle?

Systemic symptoms

+ **Constitutional** – Have you recently been unwell with a flu-like illness? Do you feel tired? Have you noticed any weight loss? How is your appetite?
+ **Lymphadenopathy** – Have you noticed any lumps in your neck or elsewhere?
+ **Arthralgia/myalgia** – Any aches and pains in your joints or muscles?
+ **Infections** – Do you frequently get infections? Any infections recently?
+ **Meningitis** – Any neck stiffness or headache?

ICE

+ Have you got any idea what might be causing the bruises? Is there anything you are particularly concerned about?

PMH

+ Do you suffer from any medical conditions?
+ *Ask specifically about blood disorders and previous malignancy*

DH

+ What medications do you currently take?
+ *Ask specifically about warfarin, aspirin and clopidogrel*
+ Do you have any allergies?

FH

+ Do any conditions run in your family?
+ *Ask specifically about easy bruising and blood disorders*

SH

+ Do you drink alcohol? How much do you drink in a week? How long has this been the case? *If required, take more detailed alcohol history*
+ Do you smoke? How many cigarettes do you smoke a day? For how long have you smoked?
+ Do you use any recreational drugs?

Important points

+ In children, you must consider the possibility of non-accidental injury and safeguarding issues, including possibly interviewing the child alone. In adults, domestic abuse might still be a possibility. Truncal bruising is less likely to be due to accidental trauma
+ Petechiae aren't necessarily pathological on the head/neck after vomiting
+ In the drug history, don't forget about over-the-counter and herbal remedies which can alter platelet function and coagulation factor levels. Pay particular attention to aspirin, steroids and warfarin. Also, has a warfarinised patient been taking antibiotics recently?
+ A bleeding tendency can be the presenting feature of liver disease, so a good alcohol history is required

Differential diagnosis

Simple uncomplicated trauma

+ Bruise preceded by an obvious trauma of appropriate force with local tenderness
+ Common locations include the anterior aspect of lower legs and the forearms
+ Less likely if the bruise is on the back, buttocks, upper arm or abdomen. It is also less likely benign if found in a child less than 9 months old (less mobile)

Thrombocytopaenia

+ Many causes, including bone marrow failure, hypersplenism, haematological malignancy, uraemia and autoimmune disorders
+ Poor platelet function often results in petechiae and mucosal bleeding
+ Lymphadenopathy and recurrent infections may suggest leukaemia

Haemophilia A and B

+ Defects of factors VIII and IX, respectively; usually presents in childhood
+ Hallmark symptoms of haemarthroses and muscle haematomas
+ Severity depends on the level of functioning factor VIII/IX

Von Willebrand's disease

+ This is the most common inheritable bleeding tendency, affecting up to 1% of people. It is inherited in an autosomal dominant fashion
+ Patients mainly complain of mucosal bleeding, although prolonged bleeding after surgery isn't uncommon

Senile purpura
- Advanced age results in a decreased level of collagen, predisposing to bruising
- The bruises here are typically large and dark. The overlying skin is thin and fragile. These are usually found on extensor surfaces and forearms

Vitamin K deficiency
- In a newborn child, this should be considered
- It is possible that the child may not have been given vitamin K after birth
- In adults, due to liver disease or malabsorption with features of jaundice, history of alcohol abuse, steatorrhoea and weight loss

Collagen abnormality
- Abnormalities of the vessel walls and surrounding tissues can predispose to bleeding, e.g. Ehlers–Danlos or Marfan's syndrome
- Skeletal involvement, cardiac involvement and ophthalmological involvement
- Features include hyperextendable joints, tall stature and excess skin elasticity

Henoch-Schönlein purpura
- Typically affects younger children with a preceding URTI
- The rash looks very similar to bruises and starts on the back of the legs and buttocks or anywhere pressure is exerted, such as sock tops. There may be associated abdominal pain, bloody diarrhoea, joint pain and in severe cases symptoms of renal failure

Non-accidental injury
- In context of a paediatric history – history incompatible with child's developmental age; 'old' bruises, limp, scald/burn marks suggest NAI
- Must involve paediatric consultant if suspicion arises, who will then involve social services – all part of safeguarding team

Mongolian blue spot
- Birthmark frequently misdiagnosed as possible NAI
- Key is that mark has been present since birth

Investigations
- FBC, LFTs, clotting and blood smear
- Bleeding time
- Mixing studies and factor + inhibitor assay
- Platelet antibody assay
- Bone marrow biopsy
- Urine analysis

Management
- Haematological malignancy – urgent referral to specialist services
- NAI – involvement of seniors and social services
- HSP – supportive treatment

◆ Immune thrombocytopaenic purpura is managed according to symptoms and monitored platelet levels; oral prednisolone or immunoglobulins in flare-ups; consider splenectomy in chronic relapsing cases
◆ Haemophilia A and B – recombinant factors VIII and IX, respectively
◆ Vitamin K deficiency – IM vitamin K injections

Surgery

Abdominal pain. 34
Lumps, bumps and swellings. 38
Weight loss 41
Jaundice. 44
Claudication 47

Abdominal pain

HPC

O'SOCRATES

- **Open question** – I believe that you are suffering from pains in your tummy. Can you tell me a bit more about your problem?
- **Site** – Where exactly do you get this pain? Can you point to it precisely? Where did the pain first manifest? Has it moved?
- **Onset** – When did this pain start? *Minutes, hours, days, weeks, months?*
- **Character** – What does the pain feel like? *You may need to provide examples, such as cramping, aching, sharp, knife-like, dull, twisting, excruciating, like an electric shock, etc.*
- **Radiation** – Does the pain move anywhere else? Can you show me? Does it go into your back/around the side/groin/testicles? Do you get shoulder-tip pain?
- **Associated features** – *see below*
- **Timing** – Is the pain there all the time or does it come and go? What is the periodicity if any (*length of time the pain is present and how long between bouts*)? Is there any particular time where you have noticed you get the pain (*day, night, mealtimes, menses*)? Have you ever had this pain before? If so, what happened?
- **Exacerbating/relieving factors** – What, if anything, brings the pain on? Does anything make it worse? Does anything make it better? Have you taken anything to relieve the pain? Is it getting better/worse with time? Does body position make a difference?
- **Severity** – If you had to rate the pain from 1 to 10, with 10 being the worst pain you can imagine, how would you score this pain currently? How would you score it at its worst? How have your symptoms affected your day-to-day life?

Systems review

At this point, you need to tailor the history to the patient in front of you and use your clinical knowledge to ask more in-depth questions about the systems that could be implicated in the pathology behind the patient's symptoms. Below are some useful quick screening questions; if a positive answer is given to any of them, this necessitates further questioning about the symptom in question.

- **GIT** – Have you noticed any weight loss? How has your appetite been? Have you had any difficulty swallowing? Any heartburn? Any vomiting? *If so*, have you noticed any blood in the vomitus? Any change in your bowel motions? Any blood or mucus in your stools?
- **GUT** – How have your waterworks been? Have you noticed any blood in the urine? Any pain when passing urine? Are you going more frequently? How have your periods been (*if relevant*)? When was your last period? How regular are they?
- **CVS** – Do you ever get chest pain? Does this pain come on during exercise?

ICE

◆ Do you have any idea what might be causing your symptoms? Is there anything you are particularly concerned about or would like to discuss?

PMH

◆ Do you suffer from any medical conditions?
◆ *Ask specifically about peptic ulcer disease. inflammatory bowel disease, diverticular disease, chronic pancreatitis, gallstones, GORD, diabetes, IHD (ACS can present as upper abdominal pain)*

DH

◆ Are you currently taking any medications?
◆ *Ask specifically about steroids, NSAIDs, self-medication and recreational drugs*
◆ Do you have any allergies?

FH

◆ Do any conditions run in the family (e.g. IBD)?
◆ Has anyone else in your family suffered from this kind of pain? Were they diagnosed?

SH

◆ Do you drink alcohol? How much do you drink in a week?
◆ Do you smoke? How many cigarettes do you smoke a day? For how many years? (*Number of packets a day × years smoked = 'pack-years', which approximates total cigarette consumption*)

Important points

◆ After taking a history of the pain, you must consider differentials in your mind and ask relevant questions about the systems involved
◆ Make sure that you ask about relevant red-flag symptoms (e.g. weight loss, dysphagia, melaena and haematemesis in epigastric pain)
◆ Never forget that ACS can present as abdominal pain and, as such, relevant questions must be asked to rule this out

Differential diagnosis

The commonest causes of abdominal pain are:
◆ Constipation – often mimicking subacute obstruction
◆ Menstrual pain
◆ Appendicitis – commonest cause of acute abdominal pain presenting to A&E
◆ UTI – one of the commonest organic causes of abdominal pain in primary care
◆ Irritable bowel syndrome – a diagnosis of exclusion
◆ Non-specific pain

Whilst it is true to say that most abdominal pain is inconsequential, the danger in considering such a list is that an important diagnosis may be missed without taking a good, accurate history. It is therefore valuable to divide abdominal pain into acute presentation and chronic conditions and consider the most likely diagnoses that may present with pain in that area (*see* Figure 1).

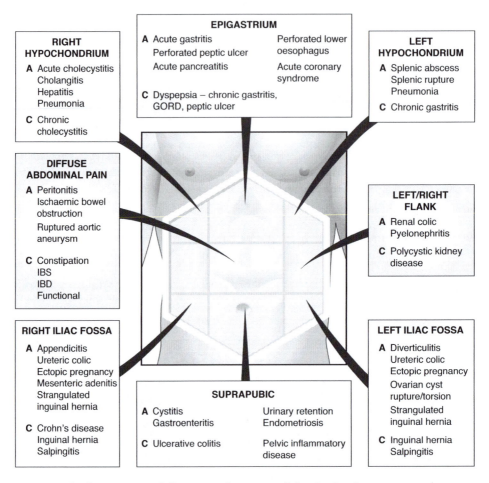

FIGURE 1 The key areas and diagnoses for acute abdominal pain

The pathophysiology of abdominal pain may be divided into parietal, visceral and referred. Parietal or somatic pain is well localised and due to local inflammation as a consequence of infection, irritation, etc. Visceral pain is usually due to distension of a viscus and is poorly localised. Pain relates to the embryonic origin of the structure, so upper-abdominal pain usually reflects stomach, duodenal, gall bladder, liver or pancreas pathology; central abdominal pain reflects those areas supplied by the superior mesenteric artery, i.e. small bowel, appendix and proximal colon; lower-abdominal pain reflects pathology in the lower colon and genitourinary tract. Referred pain is usually secondary to cardiopulmonary conditions, but may also be secondary to abdominal wall problems such as herpes zoster or muscle haematoma.

Acute abdominal pain

Acute abdominal pain almost always has a definitive pathophysiology, and it is this group that requires the most attention in terms of urgent diagnosis. In general, diagnosis and treatment are carried out simultaneously, with the key object being to rule out the most critical diagnoses where time to treatment is of the essence.

There are several diagnoses that require immediate management. These include ruptured aortic aneurysm, torsion of the testis, ectopic pregnancy, spontaneous intra-abdominal haemorrhage, acute mesenteric ischaemia and strangulated bowel. All of these have a vascular compromise. Most other acute abdominal conditions benefit from a period of stabilisation before definitive management.

Chronic abdominal pain

Chronic abdominal pain is pain which has been present for more than 6 months. There is a multitude of possible causes. Essentially, they may be divided into organic and functional aetiology, although functional is sometimes a convenient description for any abdominal pain for which no cause can be found. Up to 25% of the normal adult population will have chronic abdominal pain.

Investigations

+ Bloods – FBC, U&Es, LFTs, amylase and glucose
+ Urinalysis
+ Pregnancy test (where relevant)
+ Radiological assessment (*see below*)

With the exception of a significantly raised amylase or high glucose, blood tests are generally unhelpful and non-specific. A focused assessment with sonography for trauma (FAST) scan in A&E can pick up an aortic aneurysm, gallstones, ovarian pathology and ectopic pregnancy. The most valuable investigation (although often overused) is CT scanning.

Severity (although subjective) is important, as certain features would indicate immediate admission, e.g. 'the worst pain of my life', 'almost passed out', no bowel movement for 3 days, unable to move, pain and vomiting for > 6 hours.

It is important to remember that the result of any investigation must be considered in the light of the obtained history and subsequent examination. For example, there is a false negative rate of at least 10% in CT scans.

Lumps, bumps and swellings

In an OSCE, a history of a swelling or lump is a relatively straightforward exercise, although there are a few important factors to clarify. Most of the OSCE will probably be taken up with your examination. Typical cases will include neck lumps, abdominal swellings/masses such as hernias (commonly inguinal or incisional), polycystic disease (renal mass), simple lumps such as lipomas, chronic conditions such as neurofibromatosis, etc. Musculoskeletal lumps are also possible and often chronic (e.g. ganglions, cysts). However, you will be expected to exclude the possibility of a more serious diagnosis, particularly if the lump or swelling is in the abdomen.

HPC

O'SOCRATES

- **Open question** – I understand that you have developed a lump on your (e.g.) back. Would you like to tell me about it?
- **Site** – Where exactly is the lump? Can you point to it precisely?
- **Onset** – When did you first notice the lump? Days, weeks, months?
- **Character** – Is it there all the time? What did you first notice about it? Has it changed at all since you first noticed it?
- **Radiation** – Are there any other similar lumps that you have noticed?
- **Associated features** – Is it painful? Does it interfere with doing things?
- **Timing** – Is it there all the time or does it come and go? Is the lump more noticeable at any specific time/doing any particular activity? Have you ever had this lump/a similar lump before? *If so*, what happened?
- **Exacerbating/relieving factors** – What, if anything, makes the lump appear? Does anything make it more prominent? Does anything make it go away? Does body position make a difference (e.g. lying down)?
- **Size** – Is it getting bigger/smaller?

Systems review

Below are some useful quick screening questions; if a positive answer is given to any of them, this necessitates further questioning about the symptom in question.

- **RS** – Have you noticed a cough recently? *If so*, do you bring anything up? Any blood? Have you found yourself more breathless than previously?
- **GIT** – Have you noticed any weight loss? How has your appetite been? Have you had any difficulty swallowing? Any pain in your tummy? Any heartburn? Any vomiting? *If so*, have you noticed any blood in the vomitus? Any change in your bowel motions? Any blood in your stools?
- **GUT** – How are your waterworks? Have you noticed any blood in the urine? Any pain when passing urine? Are you going more frequently? How have your periods been (*if relevant*)?
- **MS** – Have you had any aches or pains in your muscles, bones or joints? Are your joints stiff in the morning? *If so*, for how long?

ICE

♦ Do you have any idea what might be causing your symptoms? Is there anything you are particularly concerned about or would like to discuss?

PMH

♦ Do you suffer from any medical conditions?
♦ Ask specifically about:
  ● Neck lumps – hyper- or hypothyroidism
  ● Abdominal lumps/swelling – previous surgery (e.g. incisional hernias), polycystic disease
  ● Limb or joint swelling/lumps: rheumatoid arthritis, osteoarthritis, varicose veins (saphena varix)

DH

♦ Are you taking any medications?
♦ Do you have any allergies?

FH

♦ Do any conditions run in the family? (e.g. lipomatosis, neurofibromatosis)
♦ Has anyone else in your family suffered from similar problems?

SH

♦ Do you smoke? How many cigarettes do you smoke a day? For how long have you smoked?
♦ Do you drink alcohol? How much do you drink in a week?
♦ Has anyone at home or at work been ill with anything recently? *If so, specify*

Important points

♦ This is likely to be a combined history and examination station, in which most of the time will be spent on the examination aspect. If given sufficient time for a history, you may wish to enquire about every aspect of the history, but in most cases it will suffice to ask about the characteristics of the lump (the O'SOCRATES part of the history)
♦ Always consider whether the lump could represent a malignancy and ask relevant questions to help determine the likelihood of this (e.g. weight loss, non-tender, previous cancer, high pack-year history, etc.)

Differential diagnosis

It is impossible to encompass here a complete differential diagnosis for lumps (which could be anywhere and almost anything) prior to a specific examination; however, *in the context of an OSCE* and where there is a real-life patient, the diagnoses listed below are perhaps the more common presentations. Rare conditions are only deemed so with reference to the OSCE environment.

Neck
Commonly:
- Thyroid
- Parotid
- Lymph node(s)

Rarely:
- Branchial cyst
- Cystic hygroma
- Carotid body tumour
- Thyroglossal cyst
- Carcinoma

Abdomen
Commonly:
- Inguinal hernia
- Incisional hernia
- Para/umbilical hernia
- Polycystic disease (kidney, pancreatic)

Rarely:
- Carcinoma
- Abdominal aortic aneurysm

Anywhere
- Lipoma
- Lymph node
- Neuroma

Limbs
Commonly:
- Joint cyst
- Fluid in joint
- Ganglion

Rarely:
- Bone cyst
- Tumour

Investigations and management
It is important to remember that the result of any investigation must be considered in the light of the obtained history and subsequent examination. Therefore, the investigation of a lump ranges from doing nothing (a simple lipoma) to detailed cytology following fine-needle aspiration (many neck lumps).

Likewise, the management of a lump depends on the clinical scenario. Not all lumps need to be removed and clinical acumen must be used.

Weight loss

Weight loss is a common but non-specific presentation in patients. It may represent the first manifestation of a potentially serious condition or be nothing more than an external manifestation of anxiety or depression. Excessive, unintentional weight loss is often known as cachexia (e.g. cancer cachexia, cardiac cachexia, etc.; from the Greek *kakor* – poor condition). In children, the term marasmus (from the Greek *marasmus* – wasting) is occasionally used, generally depicting a protein-deficient condition due to malabsorption. A careful, structured history will help elicit the underlying pathology. For this topic, O'SOCRATES is not a useful pneumonic, and a more basic structure is more valuable.

HPC
* **Open question** – Can you tell me what you have noticed?
* **Amount** – How much weight have you lost? Have you actually weighed yourself?
* **Onset/duration** – Over what period of time has this occurred?
* **Intentional/non-intentional** – Was this weight loss intentional or not?
* **Appetite** – How has your appetite been? Have you been eating normally or have you been on a diet?
* **Exercise** – Have you been exercising more than usual?
* **Associated features** – Have you had any recent episodes of fever or sweating, especially at night?

Systems review
Below are some useful quick screening questions; if a positive answer is given to any of them, this necessitates further questioning about the symptom in question.
* **RS** – Have you noticed a cough recently? *If so*, do you bring anything up? Any blood? Have you found yourself more breathless than previously?
* **GIT** – Have you had any difficulty swallowing? Any pain in your tummy? Any heartburn? Any vomiting? *If so*, have you noticed any blood in the vomitus? Any change in your bowel motions? Any blood in your stools?
* **GUT** – How are your waterworks? Have you noticed any blood in the urine? Any pain when passing urine? Are you going more frequently? How have your periods been (*if relevant*)?
* **NS** – Have you had any weakness in any of your muscles? Any pins and needles or strange sensations? Any headaches? Any problems with your vision or other senses?
* **MS** – Have you had any aches or pains in your muscles, bones or joints? Are your joints stiff in the morning? *If so*, for how long?

ICE
* What do you think is wrong? Is there anything you are particularly worried about? Is there anything specific that you want the doctor to help you with? How does this affect you day to day?

PMH

- Do you suffer from any medical conditions?
- *Ask specifically about recent illness, thyrotoxicosis, diabetes, chronic infections, IBD and previous cancer*

DH

- Are you taking any medications? Have any of these been changed recently?
- Do you have any allergies?

FH

- Do any specific conditions run in your family?

SH

- How much alcohol do you drink?
- Do you smoke? How many do/did you smoke a day? For how long?
- Do you take any recreational drugs?
- Are you in work/employed? What effect has this had on your job?
- Who is at home? Who cooks for you? How many meals a day?

Important points

- Useful questions include asking about clothes which no longer fit or asking if they have had to start using a belt for their trousers
- A good systems review is key to this history, as the presenting complaint can be attributed to many different systems
- Try to estimate how much weight has been lost and if it has been recent
- Ask when the patient actually last weighed themselves to gain an idea of reliability

Differential diagnosis

Weight loss is due to either inadequate intake, malabsorption, reduced anabolism, increased catabolism or a combination. Essentially, if calories used up exceed intake, then weight loss will occur. Increased catabolism is common in acute and chronic infections, but is also seen in malignancy, inflammatory conditions and post-surgery. Surgical sieves (e.g. CANDITIME – below) can be useful ways of reciting causes of any given condition, particularly for non-specific symptoms such as weight loss.

Congenital (failure to thrive)

- Genetic or chromosomal abnormalities, e.g. Down syndrome and cystic fibrosis
- Constitutional
- Others (*see* Failure to thrive – history, p. 183)

Acquired *see rest below*

Neoplasm
- Primary malignancy
- Secondary malignancy
- Benign (less likely in case of weight loss)

Degenerative
- COPD
- Multiple sclerosis

Infection/inflammatory
- Viral –short coryzal illness or more chronic infection (e.g. CMV, EBV or HIV)
- Bacterial (e.g. streptococcal pneumonia)
- Fungal (e.g. cryptococcal pneumonia)
- Other infection (e.g. TB)
- Inflammatory conditions – CTD (e.g. SLE), RA, IBD or vasculitis

Trauma (less likely cause for weight loss)

Iatrogenic/idiopathic
- Recent major surgery (e.g. gastrectomy)

Miscellaneous
- Anorexia nervosa
- Depression and/or other psychiatric diagnoses

Endocrine
- Hyperthyroidism

Investigations
- Physical examination of all systems
- Bloods – FBC, U&Es, LFTs, glucose, TFTs, CRP and ESR
- Urinalysis
- Chest X-ray
- CT scan (area depending upon clinical suspicion)

The investigation of weight loss is difficult, as the potential causes are multiple. The above is a rough guide, but clinical judgement is important to determine what other tests are important, and indeed if the above tests are all necessary.

Jaundice

Jaundice (or icterus) is a term used to describe the yellow pigmentation of a patient's skin and sclerae caused by excess bilirubin in the blood. Jaundice normally becomes visible at bilirubin levels above 35 μmol/L. An OSCE station may have either a simulated patient or perhaps a patient with long-standing jaundice from whom a focused history is required.

HPC
O'SOCRATES

- **Opening question** – I understand that you have noticed that your skin/eyes is/are a bit yellow. Would you like to tell me about it?
- **Site** – Where did you/others first notice the yellow colour (eyes/face/trunk)?
- **Onset** – When was the first time you (or someone else) noticed you were yellow?
- **Character/progression** – Is it getting worse? Does it come and go?
- **Radiation** – Has your urine become dark?
- **Associated symptoms** – *see later*
- **Timing** – How long have you noticed that you have been yellow? Has this ever happened before? How long has this been going on for?
- **Exacerbating factors** – Is the jaundice made worse by anything (e.g. foods)?
- **Severity** – When was the jaundice at its worst, do you think?

Associated symptoms

Do you have/have you had _____?
- **Loss of appetite or weight loss**
- **Dark urine**
- **Skin itching (pruritis)** – *this often begins before the jaundice*
- **Pain** – *if so, SOCRATES*
- **Pale stools**
- **Fever and fatigue/malaise**
- **Rash**
- **Confusion**
- **Abdominal swelling**

Alcohol screening history (including CAGE questionnaire)

- How much alcohol do you drink in a week? Is this a typical week for you? Do you ever binge on alcohol? *If so*, how often do you tend to binge?
- **Cut down** – Have you ever felt you should cut down on your drinking?
- **Annoyed** – Have other people ever annoyed you by commenting on your drinking?
- **Guilt** – Have you ever felt guilty about the amount you drink?
- **Eye-opener** – Have you ever had a drink in the morning to settle yourself?

If answered yes to any of the CAGE questions, take a full alcohol history (*see* p. 144).

ICE
+ Do you have any idea what might be causing your symptoms? Is there anything you are particularly concerned about or would like to discuss?

PMH
+ Do you suffer from any medical conditions?
+ Have you ever been jaundiced before?
+ Have you ever had a blood transfusion?
+ *Ask specifically about gallstones, hepatitis, pancreatitis, previous cancer and surgery and autoimmune disorders*

DH
+ Do you take any regular medications? Have any of them been changed recently?
+ Do you have any allergies?

FH
+ Do any conditions run in your family?
+ Any family history of jaundice?

SH
+ Do you smoke? How many cigarettes do you smoke a day? For how long have you smoked?
+ Have you ever used recreational drugs or self-injected?
+ Have you been abroad recently/in the past? *If so*, where?
+ Has anyone else had jaundice recently who you know/have met?

Important points
+ It is very important to take a good alcohol history, as alcohol is one of the commonest pathological causes of jaundice
+ Consider whether the patient has simply been unwell recently with a viral illness – Gilbert's syndrome is the commonest cause of jaundice and tends to be more pronounced during periods of illness

Differential diagnosis
Jaundice is usually classified as pre-hepatic, hepatic or post-hepatic, and a good history should establish which of these is most likely to be the underlying cause. Remember, jaundice may occasionally reflect a combination of both hepatic and post-hepatic causes. The key to the OSCE history is to identify whether the jaundice is pre-, intra- or post-hepatic and then to isolate the most likely aetiology. The differential diagnosis for jaundice is vast.

Pre-hepatic jaundice
+ Congenital hyperbilirubinaemia, e.g. Gilbert's syndrome and Crigler–Najjar syndrome

+ Excess production or failure of uptake into liver
+ Haemolysis, e.g. G6PD deficiency

Hepatocellular jaundice
+ Alcoholic hepatitis
+ Viral hepatitis A, B and C, EBV
+ Drug-induced hepatitis
+ Autoimmune hepatitis
+ Cirrhosis
+ Hepatocyte failure/damage
+ Hepatocellular carcinoma
+ Metastases
+ Hepatoma
+ Wilson's
+ Hepatic congestion from cardiac failure

Cholestatic jaundice
+ Impaired excretion of bile (ALP > ALT)
+ Gallstones
+ Head of pancreas cancer
+ Porta hepatis lymph nodes
+ Primary biliary sclerosis
+ Sclerosing cholangitis

Claudication

HPC

O'SOCRATES

- **Open question** – Can you tell me about the pain?
- **Site** – Where do you get the pain? (buttock, thigh, calf)
- **Onset** – Did it come on suddenly or gradually?
- **Character** – What does it feel like? (cramping, tightening of muscles)
- **Radiation** – Does the pain go anywhere else?
- **Associated factors** – Do you get any pain at night? Have you noticed any ulcers in your legs or feet? *If so*, are they painful?
- **Timing** – Do you get the pain when walking or at rest? Any previous episodes and interventions?
- **Exacerbating & relieving factors** – Is it relieved by rest? Is it made worse if you walk faster or up a hill? Does cold weather affect it?
- **Severity** – How badly does it affect you? How far can you walk before stopping? Do you want to have something done about it?

ICE

- What do you think is causing this? What is your biggest concern? Are you worried about anything else?

PMH

- Do you suffer from any medical conditions?
- *Ask specifically about diabetes, previous stroke and heart attacks, hypertension and hypercholesterolaemia*

DH

- Are you taking any medications?
- Do you have any allergies?
- *Ask specifically about blood pressure drugs, aspirin, statins, warfarin*

FH

- Do any conditions run in the family?
- *Ask specifically about diabetes, stroke and vascular disease*
- Causes of mother's and father's death

SH

- Do you smoke? (Have you ever smoked?) How many do/did you smoke? How many years have you smoked/did you smoke for?
- Does anybody else in the house smoke?
- Do you drink alcohol? How much do you drink?
- Are you still in work/employed? What effect has the problem had on your job/life?
- Who is at home? Do you have stairs? Have you had any modifications put in place, such as rails or a chairlift?

Important points

◆ Claudication pain does not occur at rest, sitting or lying down – check that the patient never gets this particular pain except when walking

◆ Older patients may have other exercise-limiting conditions (such as dyspnoea), so be certain to establish which the more significant problem is for them

◆ Use medications as a way of cross-checking the patient's medical history (they will often forget to mention hypertension, as they consider this to be under control!)

Differential diagnosis

Peripheral vascular disease

◆ Claudication pain is a cramping pain in the calf, thigh or buttocks

◆ Brought on by exercise and relieved by rest (patients often pretend to 'window-shop' until the pain disappears)

◆ Exacerbated by walking faster or up hills and also by cold weather

◆ Risk factors/associated factors for atherosclerosis:
  ● Diabetes
  ● Hypercholesterolaemia
  ● Stroke
  ● Ischaemic heart problems (myocardial infarction/angina)
  ● Hypertension
  ● Arrhythmias

◆ Rest pain may indicate critical limb ischaemia

Osteoarthritis

◆ Pain localised to feet, ankles, or knees (i.e. joints)

◆ Often pain elsewhere, e.g. hands and neck

◆ Very common; often coexists

Sciatica

◆ Shooting pain down the back of a leg to the feet

◆ History of lower-back pain

Deep vein thrombosis

◆ Tender, swollen, warm and red leg

◆ Risk factors: immobilisation, pregnancy, cancer, combined oral contraceptive pill

Spinal claudication

◆ Often relieved when walking up a hill

◆ Often has associated limb numbness

◆ Relatively uncommon

Musculoskeletal injury
+ History of preceding injury
+ Localised pain and tenderness

Investigations
+ Full peripheral vascular, cardiovascular and neurological examination
+ Assess gait and balance
+ Bloods – FBC, U&Es, biochemical profile, glucose, cholesterol (HDL/LDL)
+ ECG
+ Blood pressure – both arms (asymptomatic subclavian artery occlusion is quite common and will give a low blood pressure)
+ Ankle brachial pressure indices (Doppler-derived)
+ Duplex scan of common femoral and superficial femoral arteries
+ Establish whether proximal ('inflow') aortoiliac disease or more distal ('outflow') superficial femoral/popliteal disease, or both

Management
+ Stop smoking – firm counselling is needed, with the emphasis on taking responsibility for their health; complete cessation is the aim ('slowing down' does not work)
+ Exercise (walking)
+ Point out alternative ways of getting from A to B (bus, cycling, car, etc.)
+ Start secondary risk-prevention measures (e.g. statin, aspirin)
+ Unless patient has severe disease, consider a trial of conservative management and review in 6 months
+ If intervention (e.g. angioplasty or bypass graft) is to be considered, then an angiogram will be needed – be aware of risk of metformin and ionising contrast media (possible renal failure)

Cardiorespiratory medicine

Chest pain 52
Breathlessness 56
Palpitations 60
Cough 63
Haemoptysis 66

Chest pain
HPC
O'SOCRATES
+ **Open question** – Can you tell me about your pain?
+ **Site** – Where exactly is the pain? Can you point to where it is?
+ **Onset** – When did it start? Did it come on suddenly or gradually? What were you doing at the time?
+ **Character** – How would you describe the pain?
+ **Radiation** – Does the pain go anywhere?
+ **Associated factors** – *see later*
+ **Timing** – Is the pain always there or does it come and go? What brings the pain on? Have you ever had this pain before?
+ **Exacerbating/relieving factors** – Does anything make the pain better or worse? Is it worse when you walk? Does it go away with rest? Is there any relation to eating food? Is it better when you are in any particular position, e.g. sitting up? Is it worse when taking deep breaths?
+ **Severity** – How bad is the pain on a scale of 1–10, with 10 being the worst pain you can imagine? How would you score it at its worst?

Associated features
+ **Nausea/sweating/doom** – Do you feel sick with the pain? Have you been sweating much since it started?
+ **Breathlessness** – Do you get breathless?
+ **Orthopnoea** – Do you ever get breathless when lying flat? How many pillows do you sleep with at night?
+ **Paroxysmal nocturnal dyspnoea** – Do you ever wake up gasping for breath?
+ **Palpitations** – Do you ever get palpitations or an awareness of your heart beating? *If so*, are they fast, slow, regular or irregular?
+ **Cough** – Have you noticed a cough? Do you bring anything up? Any blood?
+ **Constitutional** – Have you noticed any weight loss? How is your appetite?
+ **Musculoskeletal** – Is the pain worse on movement? Does it hurt to press on the area?

ICE
+ What do you think is causing this? What is your biggest concern? Are you worried about anything else?

PMH
+ Do you suffer from any medical conditions?
+ *Ask specifically about angina, diabetes, hypertension and GORD*
+ **PE risk factors** – Do you have any clotting disorders? Have you ever had cancer? Any recent surgery? Have you been on any long-haul flights recently?

DH

+ Do you take any regular medications, creams, sprays or pills?
+ Do you have any allergies?

FH

+ Do any conditions run in the family?
+ Is there any family history of heart disease? *If so, clarify the ages of onset in any immediate family members*
+ *Otherwise, ask specifically about hypercholesterolaemia, hypertension and diabetes*

SH

+ Do you smoke? (Have you ever smoked?) How many do/did you smoke? How many years have you smoked/did you smoke for?
+ Do you drink alcohol? How much do you drink in a week?
+ Are you currently employed? *If so*, what do you do for a living? How has this affected your job?

Important points

+ The patients most likely to appear are those with stable angina, a previous history of ACS, GORD or musculoskeletal pain
+ The first important point to clarify is whether or not this is an acute event, as this will push the diagnosis towards a more sinister cause
+ Cardiac pain is often dull and described as 'tightness', 'discomfort' or 'a dull weight'. 'Sharp' pain is more likely parietal than visceral, i.e. decreased probability of ACS
+ Pleuritic pain (typically a sharp pain that is worse on breathing in) is less suggestive of IHD, and more of PE, pericarditis, pneumonia or costochondritis
+ Reflux tends to be a burning pain (when describing the pain, the patient typically makes a fist and presses it up and down against his or her sternum)
+ Breathlessness, orthopnoea and paroxysmal nocturnal dyspnoea indicate heart failure
+ Onset of heart disease in immediate family members before the age of 55 years in men and 65 years in women is a positive family history

Differential diagnosis

Think of cardiac causes in patients over the age of 50. Similarly, unless there is a family history, consider other causes in younger patients.

Acute coronary syndrome

+ Sudden severe crushing central pain that may radiate to the arm and/or jaw
+ Associated breathlessness, nausea, vomiting and sweating
+ Typically an old, obese male smoker with a sedentary lifestyle
+ Angina often coexists, but the pain is described as different to their usual pain

Stable angina

◆ Central chest pain that may radiate to the arm and/or jaw
◆ Pain brought on by exercise and relieved by rest; no relation to food
◆ Associated breathlessness, but sweating, nausea and vomiting are not typical
◆ It is less likely to be simple angina if the pain remains after 20 minutes of rest and there is no relief from GTN spray

Aortic dissection

◆ Sudden onset of severe tearing/ripping pain felt between the shoulder blades
◆ Possible recent history of trauma including road traffic accidents, background of hypertension or Ehler–Danlos/Marfan's syndrome
◆ Wide range of secondary symptoms reflecting interruption of blood flow from the aorta. These include acute ischaemic limbs, cerebral vascular accidents or even acute myocardial infarction, just to complicate matters

Pulmonary embolism

◆ Sudden onset of pleuritic pain with associated shortness of breath, fever and haemoptysis
◆ They may have noticed a swollen, hot, tender leg unilaterally previously
◆ Risk factors include malignancy, pregnancy, clotting disorders, recent long-haul flights or surgery with subsequent immobility

Tension pneumothorax

◆ Sudden onset of pleuritic chest pain with associated shortness of breath
◆ Background history of lung disease or collagen disease such as Marfan's syndrome or recent chest trauma (including recent insertion of a central line)

Pneumonia

◆ History of cough and purulent sputum with general malaise and fever
◆ Pleuritic chest pain with haemoptysis, wheezing and shortness of breath
◆ There may be a background history of respiratory disease (e.g. COPD)

Musculoskeletal pain (including costochondritis, aka Tietze's syndrome)

◆ Localised, superficial pleuritic pain with no other associated symptoms
◆ There may or may not be a previous history of trauma
◆ Consider in younger patients with long-standing chest pain

Gastro-oesophageal reflux disease

◆ Retrosternal burning sensation, worse on lying flat, after eating large meals, bending forward or straining
◆ Relieved by swallowing saliva, water or taking antacids
◆ Associated with the sensation of some regurgitation of acid and a sour taste

Pericarditis

◆ Pleuritic pain typically felt retrosternally and aggravated by coughing
◆ Classically, the pain is better on sitting forward and worse on lying flat

Investigations

- Cardiorespiratory examination
- 12-Lead ECG – perform promptly if ACS is suspected
- Bloods – FBC, U&Es, CRP and cardiac markers (baseline and 12 hours)
- Blood cultures
- Chest X-ray
- CT scan if suspecting aortic dissection
- CTPA or V/Q scan if PE suspected
- D-dimer (if you don't suspect PE but still want to rule it out)
- Stress ECG (not in the acute setting) or myocardial perfusion scans, or coronary calcium score if available
- Angiogram
- Oesophageal manometry and pH studies
- Endoscopy

Management

- In suspected ACS, initially manage with morphine, 100% oxygen, glyceryl trinitrate, aspirin and clopidogrel (MONAC); after confirmation of ACS, PCI or thrombolysis, depending on services available locally; long-term management includes ACE inhibitors, beta blockers and statins
- Aortic dissection – IV beta blockers and nitrates initially; Stanford type A dissections require surgery; type B dissections are usually managed medically
- Tension pneumothorax – large-bore needle decompression in the second intercostal space mid-clavicular line, with subsequent chest drain placement typically fifth intercostal space mid-axillary line
- PE – low-molecular-weight heparin and warfarin commencement

Breathlessness

HPC

COF RESUS

- ◆ **Clarify** – What exactly do you mean by breathlessness?
- ◆ **Onset** – How long has this been going on for?
- ◆ **Frequency** – Are you always breathless or only sometimes? What sets it off?
- ◆ **Relieving factors** – Does anything help you get your breath back? If you rest for a while, does it improve? Do inhalers help?
- ◆ **Exacerbating factors** – Does anything make it worse? Is it worse lying flat?
- ◆ **Sleeping upright** – How many pillows do you sleep with? Do you have to prop yourself up? Do you ever wake up gasping for air?
- ◆ **Severity** – How far can you walk before the breathlessness stops you? Can you climb a flight of stairs in one go? *If not*, how many can you manage?

Associated features

- ◆ **Cough** – Have you noticed a cough? *If so*, for how long? Do you bring anything up? Have you noticed any blood?
- ◆ **Wheeze** – Do you get wheezy? Is it worse at any time of the day?
- ◆ **Fever** – Have you recently had a cough or cold? Do you have a fever?
- ◆ **Constitutional** – Have you had any weight loss? How is your appetite?
- ◆ **Chest pain** – Do you suffer from chest pain? *If so*, SOCRATES
- ◆ **Palpitations** – Do you get palpitations with the breathlessness? *If so*, are they fast, slow, regular or irregular?
- ◆ **Anxiety** – *If relevant*, do you only get breathless when you are anxious?

ICE

- ◆ What do you think is causing this? What is your biggest concern? Are you worried about anything else?

PMH

- ◆ Do you suffer from any medical conditions?
- ◆ *Ask specifically about asthma, COPD, heart disease, diabetes and hypertension (also ask about eczema and hay fever if considering asthma)*

DH

- ◆ Are you currently taking any medication?
- ◆ Do you have any allergies?

FH

- ◆ Do any conditions run in the family?
- ◆ *Ask specifically about heart disease and asthma (also ask about eczema and hay fever if considering asthma)*

SH

+ Do you smoke? How many cigarettes do you smoke a day? For how long have you smoked?
+ What is/was your job? *If relevant*, did that involve working with asbestos?
+ Tell me about your home situation. Do you cope OK? Do you need help with anything?

Important points

+ Make an attempt to quantify breathlessness. Sedentary patients complaining of breathlessness on walking to their bathroom may be more significant than an ageing athlete who can't complete a marathon any more
+ If a patient can climb the stairs in one go, they should be capable of having a lung removed without significant impairment
+ COPD is less likely if there is less than a 20-pack-year history
+ You need to assess to what extent the patient's dyspnoea affects their life. There might not be any need for aggressive intervention if their symptoms are not intrusive

Differential diagnosis

Acute/subacute

Asthma attack

+ Sudden onset of wheezing and breathlessness
+ Often precipitated by a trigger such as exercise, cold air, dust or pollen
+ Recurrent problem, often with atopic background (e.g. eczema and hay fever)
+ Diurnal variation of asthma classically causes night-time coughing

Pulmonary embolism

+ Sudden onset of pleuritic pain with breathlessness, fever and haemoptysis
+ They may have noticed a swollen, hot, tender leg unilaterally previously
+ Risk factors include malignancy, pregnancy, clotting disorders, recent long-haul flights or surgery with subsequent immobility

Tension pneumothorax

+ Sudden onset of pleuritic chest pain with associated shortness of breath
+ Background history of lung disease or collagen disease such as Marfan's syndrome or recent chest trauma (including recent insertion of a central line)

Acute coronary syndrome

+ Sudden severe crushing central pain that may radiate to the arm and/or jaw
+ May be 'silent' though, with only breathlessness, particularly in elderly
+ Associated nausea, vomiting and sweating

Pneumonia

+ History of cough and purulent sputum with general malaise and fever
+ Pleuritic chest pain with haemoptysis, wheezing and shortness of breath.
+ There may be a background history of respiratory disease (e.g. COPD)

Acute pulmonary oedema

- Severe breathlessness often precipitated by ACS, arrhythmia, or deterioration of renal function
- Orthopnoea, paroxysmal nocturnal dyspnoea and cough (frothy pink sputum)

Chronic
Chronic obstructive pulmonary disease

- Constant breathlessness, with episodes of exacerbation due to infection
- Long smoking history, with chronic cough, wheeze and sputum production
- Progressive with increasing exertional dyspnoea and increasing disability

Interstitial lung disease

- Chronic and progressive breathlessness on exertion
- Wheezing, chest pain, haemoptysis and sputum are not typically seen
- Many environmental and occupational risk factors, e.g. farmer's lung

Lung malignancy

- Weight loss and haemoptysis are red flags; significant smoking history
- Progressive breathlessness, hoarse voice, dysphagia, wheezing, stridor, recurrent chest infections and chest discomfort are all features
- Paraneoplastic syndrome also possible due to ectopic hormone production, e.g. Cushing's or SIADH – these are usually related to small-cell lung cancer

Chronic heart failure

- Exertional dyspnoea, orthopnoea and paroxysmal nocturnal dyspnoea
- Background history of heart disease (e.g. IHD or hypertension)

Investigations

- Full cardiorespiratory examination and bedside observations
- ECG
- FBC, U&Es, cardiac markers and BNP
- ABG
- Chest X-ray
- Peak flow and pulmonary function tests
- CTPA or V/Q scan if CTPA unavailable
- Echocardiography
- Coronary angiogram
- High-resolution CT of chest

Management

- ABCDE approach in acutely unwell patients
- Smoking cessation and pulmonary rehabilitation are key in the long term
- Oxygen should be given to any patient with low saturations, with target range of 94%–98% in most patients, and 88%–92% in those with COPD
- Acute asthma – 100% oxygen, nebulised salbutamol and oral/IV steroids; ipratropium, magnesium sulphate and ICU referral if poor response

◆ In suspected ACS, initially manage with morphine, 100% oxygen, nitrate (GTN spray), aspirin and clopidogrel (MONAC); after confirmation of ACS, PCI or thrombolysis, depending on services available locally; long-term management includes ACE inhibitors, beta blockers and statins
◆ Pulmonary oedema – IV furosemide and nitrate infusion
◆ COPD exacerbation – antibiotics, bronchodilators, oxygen and steroids
◆ PE – low-molecular-weight heparin and warfarin commencement
◆ Pneumonia – antibiotics; a CURB-65 score of 2 or more requires admission

Palpitations
HPC
SOCRATES
+ **Specify** – What exactly do you mean by palpitations? Can you feel your heart beating in your chest?
+ **Onset** – Do the palpitations start suddenly or gradually?
+ **Character** – When they occur, does your heart pound fast or slow?
+ **Rhythm** – Does your heart beat regularly or irregularly?
+ **Associated features** – *see below*
+ **Timing** – How long do they last for? Do they come on at a particular time? During exercise? At night? When you feel anxious? How often do you get palpitations?
+ **Exacerbating/relieving factors** – Does anything help stop the palpitations? Do they stop suddenly, gradually or only with certain manoeuvres/drugs?
+ **Severity** – Do you get the palpitations more frequently now than previously?

Differentials
+ **Cardiac** – Do you get any chest pain? Breathlessness? Any dizzy spells or faints with the palpitations?
+ **Anxiety** – Do the attacks typically follow episodes of anxiety or panic? Are you normally an anxious person?
+ **Thyrotoxicosis** – Do you find yourself feeling hot all the time? Have you lost weight recently? Do you get diarrhoea? Are your periods regular?
+ **Phaeochromocytoma** – When your palpitations occur, do you also get sweaty? Do you feel nauseous? Do you get any abdominal pain? Do you have uncontrolled high blood pressure?

ICE
+ What do you think is causing this? What is your biggest concern? Are you worried about anything else?

PMH
+ Do you suffer from any medical conditions?
+ *Ask specifically about heart disease, psychiatric history and thyroid disorders*

DH
+ Are you currently taking any medications?
+ *Ask specifically about insulin, oral hypoglycaemic medications and thyroxine*
+ Do you have any allergies?

FH
+ Do any conditions run in the family?
+ *Ask specifically about heart disease and sudden unexpected deaths*

SH
+ Do you smoke? Do you drink alcohol? Do you take any recreational drugs?
+ Do you drink much tea or coffee?
+ What is your occupation?

Important points
+ Identifying patients with a propensity to sudden cardiac death is one of the main objectives in assessing palpitation patients
+ A family history of sudden cardiac death is very significant and warrants a more urgent investigation
+ Palpitations brought on by minimal exercise/stress can be a sign of significant cardiac pathology

Differential diagnosis
Cardiac causes
Palpitations may represent an arrhythmia, but most arrhythmias do not produce palpitations. Syncope or a history of IHD makes ventricular tachycardia and other serious arrhythmias more likely, requiring more prompt investigation.

Atrial fibrillation
+ Often asymptomatic, but there may be signs and symptoms of heart failure
+ There may be a recent history of a cardiac event or major surgery
+ May be paroxysmal, persistent or permanent
+ Causes include IHD, valvular disease, thyrotoxicosis, alcohol and pneumonia

Atrio-ventricular nodal re-entry tachycardia
+ Paroxysmal palpitations and sometimes associated syncope
+ E.g. Wolff–Parkinson–White syndrome

Ventricular tachycardia
+ Often short-lived and asymptomatic, but prolonged episodes may cause haemodynamic compromise
+ Typically occurs in patients with cardiac pathology such as IHD, heart failure, cardiomyopathies or long QT syndrome
+ Family history may reveal a sudden death in a family member

Ectopic beats
+ Typically, patients feel a skipped beat, followed by an uncomfortable lurch in the chest; some patients describe an inability to catch their breath
+ The palpitations may be more evident when the patient lies flat, commonly at night-time (related to the natural slowing of the heart rate at this time)

Non-cardiac causes
Thyrotoxicosis
+ History of weight loss, heat intolerance, hair loss, altered appetite, loose bowels, tremor, neck swelling, palpitations and menstrual irregularity

Anxiety

+ History of anxiety, agitations, sweating, nausea and dry mouth
+ An intense feeling of panic or anxiety usually precedes the palpitations
+ Palpitations are often regular, slightly fast and tend to come and go gradually

Phaeochromocytoma

+ Very rare catecholamine-secreting tumour of the adrenal glands
+ Patients typically present with hypertension, sweats, palpitations and tremor
+ May be associated with multiple endocrine neoplasia type 2 (medullary thyroid carcinoma, parathyroid gland hyperplasia and phaeochromocytoma)

Investigations

+ Full cardiovascular examination
+ 12-Lead ECG
+ 24–48-hour ambulatory ECG tape (Holter monitor)
+ Transtelephonic event monitoring for less frequent attacks
+ FBC, U&Es, TFTs
+ Echocardiogram if ECG abnormal
+ Anxiety questionnaire, e.g. HAD10
+ Electrophysiological studies
+ 24-hour urine catecholamines

Management

+ Avoid substances that predispose to palpitations, such as caffeine and alcohol
+ Supraventricular tachycardias – vagal manoeuvres (e.g. carotid massage or Valsalva manoeuvre); IV adenosine if vagal manoeuvres fail; radio-frequency catheter ablation of an identified focus for long-term cure
+ Ventricular tachycardia – high-flow oxygen; if haemodynamically unstable, treat as a cardiac arrest according to ALS protocol; if stable, may initially be treated with lignocaine or amiodarone; if there is underlying structural heart disease, prophylactic medication and an implantable cardiac defibrillator should be considered
+ Thyrotoxicosis – propranolol; carbimazole/propylthiouracil; radioiodine or subtotal/total thyroidectomy (plus lifelong thyroxine) if anti-thyroid drugs fail
+ Atrial fibrillation – rate control achieved using either beta blockers or rate-limiting calcium channel blockers; rhythm control achieved using flecainide, IV amiodarone, or by DC cardioversion; if high risk of stroke, start warfarin
+ Anxiety – counselling, CBT, SSRIs or benzodiazepines for severe anxiety; symptoms can be controlled with beta blockers
+ Ectopic beats – usually no treatment required; they are not associated with a poor prognosis, and education is all that is needed to reassure patients

Cough
HPC
Timeline
+ **Onset** – When did you first notice the cough?
+ **Progression** – Has it changed recently? *If so*, in what way?
+ **Timing** – Is it there all the time? Is it worse at any particular time of the day? Does it vary with the seasons or weather?
+ **Triggers** – Does anything set the cough off? Have you inhaled anything like dust or smoke that set it off?

Associated features
+ **Sputum** – Do you cough anything up or is it a dry cough? *If so*, how much? What colour is it? Do you normally cough anything up?
+ **Blood** – Do you ever cough up blood? Is it mixed in or streaky? How long has this been going on for?
+ **Wheeze** – Have you noticed a wheeze or any other strange sounds?
+ **Breathlessness** – Have you been breathless? *If so, quantify exercise tolerance*
+ **Chest pain** – Do you have any chest pain? *If so, SOCRATES*
+ **Malaise** – Have you been feeling generally unwell with fever and chills?
+ **URTI** – Do you currently have a cold? Is your nose runny or throat sore? Do you have a headache? *If so*, is it worse on bending forwards or pressing your face? Do you have to constantly clear your throat?
+ **Weight loss** – Have you recently lost any weight? How is your appetite?
+ **Reflux** – Do you suffer from heartburn? Is your cough worse on lying flat?

ICE
+ What do you think is causing this? What is your biggest concern? Are you worried about anything else?

PMH
+ Do you suffer from any medical conditions?
+ *Ask specifically about asthma and COPD*

DH
+ Are you currently taking any medications?
+ *Ask specifically about ACE inhibitors*
+ Do you have any allergies?

FH
+ Do any conditions run in the family?
+ *Ask specifically about lung cancer, asthma and allergies*

SH
+ What is your occupation? Are you exposed to any dust or asbestos?

+ Do you smoke? How many cigarettes do you smoke a day? For how long have you smoked?
+ What is your home situation like? Have you moved home recently?

Important points
+ The occupational history is very important for a chronic cough – legal proceedings against employers are very common now, especially for conditions such as asbestosis, for which a properly documented cough history and exposure to harmful substances is vital
+ In a child, consider the possibility of an inhaled foreign body, especially where there is a prominent stridor

Differential diagnosis
Acute (<3 weeks)
Post-nasal drip
+ This is a common cause of a cough in a non-smoking adult
+ Short history of an irritating cough with a recent URTI, but otherwise well
+ Runny nose, congestion, sore throat, sinusitis and throat-clearing

Pneumonia
+ History of cough and purulent sputum production with malaise and fever
+ There may be pleuritic chest pain, haemoptysis, wheezing and breathlessness
+ Often a background history of respiratory disease (e.g. COPD/bronchiectasis)

ACE inhibitors
+ ACE inhibitors cause a dry cough in 5%–20% of patients
+ No other symptoms present
+ Usually presents within a week of starting therapy, but can be up to 6 months

Subacute (3–8 weeks)
Lung malignancy
+ Weight loss and haemoptysis are red flags; significant smoking history
+ Progressive breathlessness, hoarse voice, dysphagia, wheezing, stridor, recurrent chest infections and chest discomfort are all features
+ Paraneoplastic syndrome also possible due to ectopic hormone production, e.g. Cushing's or SIADH – these are usually related to small-cell lung cancer

Gastro-oesophageal reflux disease
+ Typically overweight patient with retrosternal burning pain worse on lying flat
+ Acid brash, with regurgitation of sour material after eating large meals
+ May have a hoarse voice in the morning and periodically clear their throat

Chronic (> 8 weeks)
Asthma
+ Diurnal variation – cough worse at night and in the morning
+ Coughing is worse in cold air or after exercise

- May be associated wheezing and breathlessness
- Often a background history of atopy, such as eczema and hay fever

Chronic obstructive pulmonary disease
- Constant breathlessness, with episodes of exacerbation due to infection
- Long smoking history, with chronic cough, wheeze and sputum production
- Progressive with increasing exertional dyspnoea and increasing disability

Bronchiectasis
- Precipitated by recurrent infections or a particularly bad chest infection
- Production of large amounts of sputum ('cupfuls') each day
- Haemoptysis and breathlessness may be present
- Cystic fibrosis is associated with bronchiectasis

Investigations
- Full cardiorespiratory examination
- FBC, U&Es, LFTs and blood culture
- Sputum culture
- Peak flow
- Chest X-ray
- Pulmonary function tests
- Bronchoscopy
- CT thorax
- Methacholine challenge

Management
- Post-nasal drip – antihistamines and a decongestant
- Pneumonia – antibiotics; a CURB-65 score of 2 or more requires admission
- Asthma – stepwise approach, starting with inhaled salbutamol PRN; regular inhaled corticosteroid may be added, and then a long-acting beta2-agonist; leukotriene antagonists, theophylline and oral steroids may also be needed
- COPD – stop smoking, inhaled bronchodilators, inhaled corticosteroids and consider long-term domiciliary oxygen therapy
- Lung cancer – urgent referral; surgery, chemotherapy and/or radiotherapy
- GORD – proton-pump inhibitor and antacids
- ACE inhibitor cough – stop and switch to angiotensin receptor blocker

Haemoptysis

- **Open question** – Can you tell me exactly what you have noticed?
- **Site** – Are you definitely coughing blood up, not vomiting it up? Is it only there when you cough or also at other times? Any recent nosebleeds? *If so, could it just be that you are coughing up blood from the nosebleed?*
- **Onset** – When did you first notice it?
- **Timing** – How many times have you noticed it?
- **Character** – What colour is it? Bright red? Dark?
- **Amount** – How much are you coughing up? Streaks or larger amounts?

HPC

Associated features

- **Cough** – Have you been coughing otherwise recently? *If so*, how long have you had a cough for? Is it there all the time?
- **Sputum** – Do you bring up any sputum? *If so*, what colour is it? How much do you bring up? Streaks or cupfuls?
- **Chest pain** – Do you have any chest pain? *If so, SOCRATES*
- **Breathlessness** – Are you short of breath? *If so*, when did this start? Do you feel breathless all the time or in certain situations, such as during exercise?
- **Heart failure** – *If breathless*, how many stairs can you manage before needing to take a break? How far can you walk? Do your ankles swell?
- **Constitutional** – Any recent weight loss? How is your appetite? Have you been feeling feverish? Any night sweats? *If so*, are they drenching?
- **Lymphadenopathy** – Have you noticed any lumps or enlarged glands?
- **PE** – Any long-haul flights recently? Recent surgery? Swollen legs? Have you suffered from blood clots in the past?
- **Travel** – Have you travelled anywhere outside the UK within the last year?

ICE

- What do you think is causing this? What is your biggest concern? Are you worried about anything else?

PMH

- Do you suffer from any medical conditions?
- *Ask specifically about cancer, bleeding disorders and clotting disorders*

DH

- Are you currently taking any medications?
- *Ask specifically about warfarin and any contraception (the Pill)*
- Do you have any allergies?

FH

- Do any conditions run in your family?
- *Ask specifically about lung cancer, clotting disorders and bleeding disorders*

SH

+ Do you smoke? How many cigarettes do you smoke a day? For how long have you smoked?
+ Do you drink alcohol? How much do you drink in a week?
+ What is your occupation?

Important points

+ Be sure to get an accurate smoking history in anyone with haemoptysis to properly assess their risk for lung cancer – if they say they don't smoke, ask if they have ever smoked and determine their pack-year history
+ It can be hard to distinguish true haemoptysis from other sources, so clarify with them that they are definitely coughing it up and ask about non-pulmonary causes, such as nosebleeds or poor dental hygiene
+ It is important to ask about risk factors for PE to rule it out in cases of haemoptysis

Differential diagnosis

Acute bronchitis

+ Few days' history of fever, malaise and cough with shortness of breath
+ Mucopurulent sputum streaked with blood

Pulmonary embolism

+ Pleuritic chest pain with shortness of breath
+ Associated fever, tachycardia and occasionally haemoptysis
+ Possible background history of a procoagulant state such as malignancy, pregnancy or antithrombin 3 deficiency
+ Similarly, there may be a history of recent air travel or operation with long periods of immobilisation. The patient may also complain of a painful swollen leg

Lung malignancy

+ Weight loss and haemoptysis are red flags for lung cancer
+ Patients may also complain of progressive breathlessness, a hoarse voice, dysphagia, wheezing or stridor, recurrent chest infections or chest discomfort
+ Risk factors include increasing age, smoking history, occupational exposure to asbestos and other hazardous industrial dusts
+ Patients may also have symptoms of a paraneoplastic syndrome such as Cushing's (central obesity, bruising, thin skin etc.), dermatomyositis or SIADH

Lung abscess

+ Production of copious amounts of bloodstained foul-smelling sputum
+ Often significant preceding pneumonia or similar seeding event, such as infective endocarditis, foreign body aspiration or trauma
+ Swinging fevers, pleuritic chest pain, cough and weight loss

Pneumonia
- Rapid onset over a day or so of shortness of breath, cough, pleuritic chest pain, fever and general malaise
- Classically, rusty-brown sputum

Tuberculosis
- Long-standing fever, malaise, lymphadenopathy and weight loss
- Classically produces night sweats
- Risk factors for infection, including immunosuppression, travel to endemic areas, alcoholism and IV drug users

Bronchiectasis
- Precipitated by recurrent infections or a particularly bad chest infection
- Production of large amounts of sputum ('cupfuls') each day
- Haemoptysis and breathlessness may be present
- Cystic fibrosis is associated with bronchiectasis

Investigations
- Look at the sputum. Is there really any blood?
- FBC, U&Es, LFTs, clotting, CRP and ESR
- D-dimer to rule out PE
- Blood cultures
- Sputum culture
- Mantoux test/QuantiFERON-TB Gold
- Chest X-ray
- CT chest
- CTPA
- Bronchoscopy

Management
- PE – high-dose low-molecular-weight heparin and warfarin
- Tuberculosis – 6 months' treatment with isoniazid and rifampicin, with the addition for the first 2 months of pyrazinamide and ethambutol
- Pneumonia – antibiotics; a CURB-65 score of 2 or more requires admission
- Lung cancer – urgent referral; surgery, chemotherapy and/or radiotherapy
- Bronchiectasis – antibiotics; mucolytics and chest physiotherapy; bronchial artery embolisation can be considered for massive haemoptysis
- Lung abscess – IV antibiotics; percutaneous drainage via CT guidance

Gastroenterology

Dysphagia 70
Haematemesis. 74
Change in bowel habit
(constipation/diarrhoea in adults) 78
Bleeding per rectum 82

Dysphagia
HPC
STOP – a solid timeline needed
+ **Solids or liquids?** – Do you have difficulty swallowing solids, fluids or both?
+ **Timing** – Is it there all the time or does it come and go?
+ **Onset** – When did this start?
+ **Progression** – Has it worsened over time?

Associated features
+ **Stuck** – Does the food get stuck in your throat when swallowing?
+ **Halitosis** – Have you noticed having bad-smelling breath recently?
+ **Lump** – Do you ever feel a lump in your throat?
+ **Gurgle** – Do you ever notice gurgling or a wet voice after swallowing?
+ **Pain** – Is there any pain when swallowing? Any chest pain?
+ **GORD/dyspepsia** – Do you ever taste acid at the back of your mouth? Heartburn? Pain in your tummy?
+ **Haematemesis** – Have you vomited at all? *If so, was there any blood?*
+ **Bowels** – Have you noticed any change in your bowels? How many times a day do you go to the toilet? Has that changed at all? Have you noticed any blood in your stools? Is it darker or more smelly than usual?
+ **Neuro** – Have you noticed any weakness anywhere? Any problems walking?
+ **Autoimmune** – Do you suffer with painfully cold hands? Dry eyes or mouth? Tight, shiny skin? Have you noticed any change in your appearance?
+ **Constitutional** – Have you had any unintentional weight loss? *If so*, how much have you lost and over how long?

ICE
+ What do you think is wrong? Is there anything you are concerned about? Is there anything in particular that you would like the doctor to do for you?

PMH
+ Do you suffer from any medical conditions?
+ *Ask specifically about neurological conditions such as multiple sclerosis and previous history of stroke and/or malignancy*
+ Have you ever, accidentally or otherwise, drunk corrosives such as bleach?

DH
+ Do you take any medications? Any over-the-counter medications?
+ *Ask specifically about NSAIDs and steroids*
+ Do you have any allergies?

FH
+ Do any conditions run in the family?
+ *Ask specifically about autoimmune conditions and congenital abnormalities*

SH
+ Do you smoke? How many do you smoke a day? For how many years?
+ Do you drink alcohol? How much do you drink in a week?
+ What do you do for a living?
+ Who do you live with?

Important points
+ Make sure you cover all of the ALARMS symptoms
+ ALARMS symptoms – if present, consider sinister causes and refer urgently
  • **Anaemia** (unexplained)
  • **Loss of weight** (unintentional)
  • **Anorexia**
  • **Recent onset of progressive symptoms**
  • **Melaena or haematemesis**
  • **Swallowing difficulty**
  • **> 55 years old**
+ It is good to get an idea straight away about how long the problem has been going on and how things are progressing – if the nature hasn't changed and it has been there for years, sinister causes are less likely
+ Untreated dysphagia can lead to malnutrition, pneumonia and even aspiration

Differential diagnosis
Neuromuscular disorders
Stroke
+ Other features include acute onset of speech impairment and limb weakness
+ High risk of aspiration, with gurgling voice after drinking
+ Risk factors include diabetes, obesity, hypertension and atrial fibrillation

Myasthenia gravis
+ Autoimmune neuromuscular disorder characterised by muscle fatiguability
+ Difficulty initiating swallowing and subsequent coughing due to aspiration
+ Other signs and symptoms include weakness, ptosis, dysarthria, shortness of breath and waddling gait

Motor neurone disease
+ Age is usually between 50 and 70 years and more commonly seen in males
+ Progressive illness associated with upper and lower motor signs
+ In progressive bulbar palsy, quiet hoarse voice and difficulties swallowing may be the first presenting symptoms

Obstructive disorders
Benign oesophageal stricture
+ Associated with chronic GORD (acid brash and retrosternal burning pain associated with food)
+ Intermittent dysphagia for solids which gradually worsens over time
+ There may be a history of corrosive ingestion, radiation exposure or trauma

Oesophageal cancer
- Progressively worsening dysphagia, initially for solids, but later also liquids
- ALARMS symptoms suggest possibility and necessitate urgent referral
- Risk factors include advanced age, male sex, smoking, high alcohol intake and chronic GORD (Barrett's oesophagus)

Oesophageal web
- Associated with odynophagia
- Either due to congenital defect or Plummer–Vinson syndrome
- Plummer–Vinson syndrome – chronic iron-deficiency anaemia with web

Pharyngeal pouch
- Sensation of lump in throat and halitosis

External oesophageal compression
- Retrosternal goitre or other mediastinal masses such as lymphomas

Oesophageal motility disorders
Achalasia
- Impaired relaxation of lower oesophageal sphincter
- Long history of intermittent dysphagia for solids more than liquids
- Retrosternal chest pain after meals and heartburn are associated features

Oesophageal spasm
- Spontaneous intermittent chest pain commonly misdiagnosed as ACS

Systemic sclerosis
- Reflux symptoms as well as tight, thickened skin causing characteristic appearance, Raynaud's phenomenon and possible lung/heart involvement

Others
- Globus pharyngeus – somatisation disorder with sensation of lump in throat; anxiety may coexist
- Tonsillitis – subacute onset of odynophagia, pharyngitis and possibly fever

Investigations
- Full neck and abdominal examination
- Bloods – FBC, U&Es, LFTs and clotting and bone profile
- Chest X-ray
- Barium swallow
- Endoscopy and biopsy
- Videofluoroscopy – assessing for aspiration
- Staging CT scan, depending on what the previous investigations reveal

Management

- 2-week referral for patients with ALARMS symptoms
- Dietician referral for further input and assessment of nutrition
- Speech and language therapy to assess safety of swallow (risk of aspiration)
- Benign stricture – slow meals and quantity, antacids and endoscopic dilatation
- Achalasia – smooth-muscle dilator and endoscopic dilatation
- Calcium channel blocker in oesophageal spasm
- Systemic sclerosis – small meals and rheumatological referral
- Psychological therapy may be of assistance to patients with globus pharyngeus

Haematemesis

HPC

O CAT RIB - Occam's CAT Retches In Blood

- **Onset** – When did this start?
- **Clarify/character** – Is the blood definitely in your vomit, and not from coughing or a nosebleed? Is it fresh red blood or coffee-grounds in nature?
- **Amount** – How much blood have you noticed? Streaks? A teaspoon? More?
- **Timing** – Has this happened before? *If so*, what happened then?
- **Retching** – Were you retching prior to vomiting up blood?
- **Indigestion** – Have you been suffering from indigestion recently? Any abdominal pain? *If so, SOCRATES*
- **Bowels** – Have you noticed any change in your bowels? How many times a day do you go to the toilet? Has that changed at all? Have you noticed any blood in your stools? Is it darker or more smelly than usual?

ALARMS - red flags

- **Anaemia** – How have your energy levels been recently?
- **Loss of weight** – Have you had any recent unintentional weight loss? *If so*, how much have you lost and over how long?
- **Appetite poor** – How has your appetite been?
- **Recent onset of progressive symptoms** – How have your symptoms progressed? Have they come on quickly or gradually?
- **Melaena**
- **Swallowing difficulty** – Have you had any difficulty swallowing recently?

ICE

- What do you think is causing this? Is there anything you are particularly concerned about or would like the doctor to do for you?

PMH

- Do you suffer from any medical conditions?
- *Ask specifically about liver disease, peptic ulcers, previous malignancy and surgery*

DH

- Do you take any regular medications? Any over-the-counter medications?
- *Ask specifically about NSAIDs, aspirin, warfarin and steroids*

FH

- Do any conditions run in the family?
- *Ask specifically about malignancy (especially gastric carcinoma) and bleeding disorders*

SH
+ Do you smoke? How many cigarettes do you smoke a day? How long have you smoked for?
+ Do you drink alcohol? How much do you drink in a week?
+ Are you suffering with stress at the moment?
+ Do you take any recreational drugs? Do you have any tattoos?
+ What do you do for a living?
+ Who do you live with? Are you coping at home?

Important points
+ Gauge from the start whether the patient is acutely unwell or if they are comfortable and able to talk after a previous episode – this will determine whether you should proceed with a full history or whether you should start a more appropriate acute-management approach
+ It is important to distinguish haematemesis from haemoptysis or a nosebleed
+ Don't forget to ask about the ALARMS symptoms
+ The colour and amount of vomitus can be used to guide potential severity and origin – coffee-ground vomit suggests a small bleed that has been exposed to gastric acid, whereas a large amount of fresh red bleeding may suggest a large haemorrhage; a small bleed that has not been exposed to gastric acid will therefore also be fresh red

Differential diagnosis
Haematemesis carries a mortality rate of 10% and is treated as a medical emergency. Consider the principle of Occam's razor here. There are many causes of haematemesis, but the simplest explanation is likely to be the correct one (e.g. oesophageal varices in a chronic alcoholic; Mallory–Weiss tear after an alcohol binge; gastric erosions or a bleeding peptic ulcer in patients on long-term anti-inflammatories)

Common causes of haematemesis
Oesophagitis
+ History of GORD (heartburn with acid brash)
+ Fresh red blood with no ALARMS symptoms

Gastric/duodenal erosion
+ History of dyspepsia
+ Associated with prolonged use of NSAIDs, steroids, SSRIs or bisphosphonates

Bleeding peptic ulcer
+ May present very unwell with peritonitis
+ History of dyspepsia, nausea and smoking
+ Associated with prolonged use of NSAIDs, steroids, SSRIs or bisphosphonates

Oesophageal varices
+ History of liver disease, possibly due to excessive alcohol consumption
+ Bleeding can be extensive and catastrophic

Oesophageal/gastric malignancy

- ALARMS symptoms – anaemia, recent weight loss, poor appetite, recent onset of progressive symptoms, melaena and swallowing difficulty
- Early satiety is another feature of gastric carcinoma

Mallory-Weiss tear

- Typically occurs after an uncontrollable bout of retching or coughing
- Fresh red blood with a history of excessive alcohol intake or eating disorders

Rarer causes

- Arteriovenous malformations – acute extensive haemorrhage; associated with hereditary haemorrhagic telangiectasia
- Boerhaave's syndrome – oesophageal rupture due to excessive vomiting or retching; severe retrosternal and abdominal pain following vomiting; alcoholism present in 40% of patients
- Iatrogenic – recent oesophageal/gastric surgery or endoscopy
- Aortoenteric fistula – very rare condition, given some credence if the patient is known to have an abdominal aortic aneurysm or aortic graft in situ

Investigations

- Check observations, perform abdominal and PR examination
- FBC, U&Es, LFTs, clotting, CRP, bone profile and group and save (if bleeding is minimal) or crossmatch between 2 and 4 units (depending on severity)
- Erect chest X-ray – free air under diaphragm indicates perforation
- Urgent upper-GIT endoscopy
- CT abdomen/chest – for all patients with aortic grafts
- Angiography may be needed if source of bleeding not found at endoscopy

Management

Haematemesis must be treated as a medical emergency. Therefore initial management should be completed in an ABCDE approach.

A   Ensure airway is patent and secured. Use suction to remove any vomiting that could compromise airway

B   Assess respiratory rate and oxygen saturations. Give high-flow 15 L oxygen via a non-rebreathe mask. Auscultate and percuss the chest

C   Assess character, rate and volume of pulse. Establish IV access and give IV fluids to maintain circulation. Monitor blood pressure

D   Assess responsiveness with AVPU. Check pupils and blood glucose

E   Expose the patient. Check from head to toe for obvious signs of haemorrhage

Always contact a senior doctor for support and ensure patients are kept nil by mouth for emergency endoscopy/surgery. Some hospitals use the Rockall score or the Glasgow–Blatchford score to stratify those with greatest need of urgent endoscopy.

Once the patient is stable, the following management can be used:

- Advice on alcohol intake and referral to alcohol specialist team for patients suffering from alcoholism
- Medication review to identify medications that could cause gastritis/ulcers such as NSAIDs, steroids, SSRIs and bisphosphonates
- Proton-pump inhibitor cover for any patients on long-term NSAIDs/steroids
- 2-week referral for patients with suspected malignancy
- Treat positive *H. pylori* patient with triple-therapy regime (usually two antibiotics and a proton-pump inhibitor), as per local protocol

Change in bowel habit (constipation/diarrhoea in adults)

HPC

O'SOCRATES

- **Open question** – Can you tell me what has been going on?
- **Specify** – When you say constipation/diarrhoea, what do you mean exactly? Do you mean you are going more/less often or the consistency has changed?
- **Onset** – When did you first notice this? Has this changed recently?
- **Character/colour** – What are the stools like? Are they watery, semi-solid or solid? Is there any blood or mucus in the stools or on the tissue paper? What colour are your stools?
- **Radiation (from upper GIT)** – Do you get any dark, foul-smelling stools?
- **Associated features** – *see below*
- **Timing** – How many times a day do you go to the toilet to pass faeces now? How often do you normally go? What are your stools normally like? Have you ever suffered from the opposite? (i.e. constipation/diarrhoea)
- **Exacerbating/relieving factors** – Does anything relieve the constipation/diarrhoea? Does anything make it worse?
- **Severity** – How badly is this affecting your day-to-day life?

BOWELS

- **Bloating** – Do you tend to suffer from bloating and flatulence?
- **Ouch!** – Are you suffering from any abdominal pain? *If so, SOCRATES*
- **Weight loss** – Have you lost any weight recently? How is your appetite?
- **Exhaustion** – How have your energy levels been?
- **Lasting urge** – Do you feel like you always need to go to the toilet, even after you've just been? Is this despite not passing very much stool? (*Tenesmus*)
- **Swallowing/upper-GIT symptoms** – Any vomiting? (*If so, ask about haematemesis.*) Any difficulties swallowing? Heartburn?

Extra-intestinal features

- **IBD** – Have you had any mouth ulcers? Fever? Painful red eye? Joint or back pain?
- **Spinal cord lesion** – We discussed back pain, but have you had any weakness in your legs? Do you find it difficult to gain an erection (*men!*)?
- **Foreign travel** – Have you been abroad anywhere recently?

ICE

- What do you think is wrong? Is there anything you are particularly concerned about or would like dealt with?

PMH

- Do you suffer from any medical conditions?
- *Ask specifically about anaemia, IBD and previous malignancy*

DH

◆ Do you take any regular medications? Any over-the-counter medications?
◆ *Ask specifically about laxatives and antidiarrhoeals such as codeine*

FH

◆ Do any conditions run in the family?
◆ *Ask specifically about IBD and malignancy (colorectal and ovarian carcinoma – and determine which relatives they were and what age they were when they were diagnosed)*

SH

◆ Do you smoke? How many cigarettes do you smoke a day? For how long have you smoked?
◆ Do you drink alcohol? How much do you drink in a week?
◆ What do you do for a living?
◆ Who do you live with? Are you coping at home?

Important points

◆ Constipation and diarrhoea can mean different things to different people – make sure that you clarify early exactly what the patient means
◆ Quantify how many times they are going to the toilet and what effect it is having on their life
◆ Never forget to ask about red-flag symptoms (e.g. cachexia, PR bleeding, anaemia and upper-GIT symptoms)
◆ In lesions affecting the caecum/ascending colon, there may be no change in bowel habit, as faecal matter in this part of the colon is liquid/semi-solid (hence unexplained anaemia must be investigated), whereas lesions in the sigmoid colon/rectum will often cause a change in bowel habit due to obstruction
◆ Family history is very important here – do not forget!
◆ Symptoms of bloating and flatulence are often reported by patients, but they are of little clinical significance
◆ Interestingly, smoking exacerbates Crohn's disease, whereas it appears to lower the risk of developing ulcerative colitis!

Differential diagnosis

Factors likely to cause constipation

◆ Diet – lack of fibre in diet, regular consumption of processed/ready-made meals and reduced water intake
◆ Lack of exercise and immobility
◆ Medication – opioids, iron supplements, amitriptyline and many more
◆ Anorectal disease, e.g. anal fissures that make defecation a painful experience

Colorectal cancer
- Age over 55 years (unless familial predisposition mentioned)
- Red-flag symptoms include cachexia, rectal bleeding, abdominal mass found and change in bowel habit lasting 6 weeks or more
- Always consider in men of any age or non-menstruating women with unexplained iron-deficiency anaemia
- Previous history of malignancy, IBD and coeliac disease

IBD
- Chronic diarrhoea with blood and mucus, and lower abdominal pain
- Fever, mouth ulcers, anorectal disease and extra-intestinal features may be present
- Consider in younger patients with above symptoms

Irritable bowel syndrome
- Commoner in women (often young) and may be related to stress or anxiety
- Associated with bloating, constipation/diarrhoea and crampy abdominal pain
- No blood in the stools or other red flags present

Gastroenteritis
- Recent history of eating uncooked/poorly prepared food and/or foreign travel
- Diarrhoea (may be watery, bloody or simply loose) and vomiting
- Household members may also be unwell with similar symptoms

Diverticular disease
- Middle-aged/elderly patients with bloody diarrhoea and pain in left iliac fossa
- Can lead to diverticulitis, with fever, nausea and vomiting
- Risk factors include obesity and low dietary fibre

Malabsorption
- E.g. due to coeliac disease, chronic pancreatitis, thyroid disease or diabetes
- Steatorrhoea (pale, offensive stools that are difficult to flush), weight loss and general malaise may accompany diarrhoea

Others
- Overflow diarrhoea after constipation with faecal impaction
- Diabetic autonomic neuropathy
- Metabolic disturbance, e.g. thyroid hormone and calcium abnormalities

Investigations
- Full abdominal examination and PR examination
- FBC – check for anaemia
- Other bloods: LFTs, U&Es , TFTs, CRP, ESR and group and save 2–4 units
- Stool culture
- Faecal occult blood test
- Abdominal X-ray

- Flexible sigmoidoscopy ± colonoscopy and upper-GIT endoscopy
- Abdominal CT scan

Management

- 2-week referral for patients with red-flag symptoms
- Correct any electrolyte abnormalities
- Advice on diet, hydration and lifestyle, and medication review for constipation
- IBS – dietary/lifestyle advice, antispasmodics, laxatives/antidiarrhoeals, and psychological therapy
- IBD – stop smoking (Crohn's); sulfasalazine (ulcerative colitis); infliximab in severe disease; surgery; steroids for flare-ups
- Gastroenteritis – rehydration; if history of foreign travel or bloody diarrhoea, consider antibiotics
- Diverticular disease – high-fibre diet and bulk-producing laxatives if no better
- Malabsorption – treat underlying cause and give nutritional supplements

Bleeding per rectum
HPC
◆ **Site** – Can I just clarify the bleeding is coming from the back passage, not the front?
◆ **Onset** – When did you first notice this?
◆ **Character/colour** – What colour is the blood? Fresh red? Coffee grounds? How much blood have you noticed? Streaks? Teaspoon? More?
◆ **Radiation (to paper/pan)** – Did you notice the blood in the pan or on the tissue paper? Is it mixed in with the stool?
◆ **Associated features** – *see later*
◆ **Timing** – Has this happened before?
◆ **Exacerbating factors** – Does anything bring it on, such as episodes of constipation? Any recent trauma to the area?
◆ **Severity/smell** – Have you noticed it to be particularly foul-smelling?

Associated features – CATS PAWS
◆ **Change in bowel habit** – What are your stools like? Any mucus? How often do you go to the toilet to pass faeces? Is this normal for you?
◆ **Abroad** – Have you been abroad recently? *If so*, where?
◆ **Tiredness** – Have you been feeling more tired than normal recently?
◆ **Swallowing/upper-GIT symptoms** – Have you been nauseous or sick? (*If so, ask about haematemesis.*) Any difficulties swallowing? Heartburn?
◆ **Pain/pruritis ani** – Have you had any pain in your tummy? *If so, SOCRATES.* Have you noticed any itching around the anus?
◆ **Anorexia** – How has your appetite been?
◆ **Weight loss** – Have you noticed any unintentional weight loss?
◆ **Systemic features** – Have you had any mouth ulcers? Fever? Painful red eye? Joint or back pain?

ICE
◆ What do you think could be wrong? I know this can be quite a scary problem, but does anything particularly concern you that you would like dealt with?

PMH
◆ Do you suffer from any medical conditions?
◆ *Ask specifically about PR HIM*
  ● Peptic ulcers
  ● Recent GIT surgery
  ● Haemorrhoids
  ● IBD and diverticulitis
  ● Malignancy

DH
◆ Do you take any regular medications? Any over-the-counter medications?
◆ *Ask specifically about laxatives and antidiarrhoeals such as codeine*

FH

- Do any conditions run in the family?
- *Ask specifically about IBD and malignancy (colorectal and ovarian carcinoma – and determine which relatives they were and what age they were when they were diagnosed)*

SH

- Do you smoke? How many cigarettes do you smoke a day? For how long have you smoked?
- Do you drink alcohol? How much do you drink in a week?
- What do you do for a living?
- Who do you live with? Are you coping at home?

Important points

- Bleeding of any nature can be particularly frightening and/or embarrassing for most patients, and therefore it is important to approach this history in a sympathetic manner – if the patient is tentative initially, help put their mind at ease, e.g. 'Often people are frightened or embarrassed to talk about these problems, but it is a common issue and it is important that it is explored, so thank you for coming in today.'
- Never forget to ask about other red-flag symptoms (e.g. cachexia, persistent change in bowel habit for 6 weeks or more, anaemia and upper-GIT symptoms)
- Family history is very important here – do not forget
- The colour of the blood and extent it is mixed in with the stool can help determine where the bleed is likely to originate from. PR bleeding from the upper GIT is partially digested, producing melaena – a dark, extremely foul-smelling stool; bleeds of anorectal pathology will be fresh red, and those in between are usually darker and mixed in with the stool
- In lesions affecting the caecum/ascending colon, there may be no change in bowel habit, as faecal matter in this part of the colon is liquid/semi-solid (hence unexplained anaemia must be investigated), whereas lesions in the sigmoid colon/rectum will often cause a change in bowel habit due to obstruction

Differential diagnosis

Anal fissure

- Fresh red blood seen in the toilet paper, not the pan
- Can be acute or chronic, with pruritis ani commonly also found
- Fissures may cause severe pain during defecation, which makes the patient reluctant to go in future, causing constipation which exacerbates the problem

Haemorrhoids

- Fresh red blood on the toilet paper or in the pan
- Associated with pruritis ani, but are rarely painful
- History of constipation and straining

Gastroenteritis

◆ Recent history of eating uncooked/poorly prepared food and/or foreign travel
◆ Diarrhoea (may be watery, bloody or simply loose) and vomiting
◆ Household members may also be unwell with similar symptoms

Diverticular disease

◆ Middle-aged/elderly patients with bloody diarrhoea and pain in left iliac fossa
◆ Can lead to diverticulitis, with fever, nausea and vomiting
◆ Risk factors include obesity and low dietary fibre

Colorectal cancer

◆ Age over 55 years (unless familial predisposition mentioned)
◆ Red-flag symptoms include cachexia, rectal bleeding, abdominal mass found and change in bowel habit lasting 6 weeks or more
◆ Always consider in men of any age or non-menstruating women with unexplained iron-deficiency anaemia
◆ Previous history of malignancy, IBD and coeliac disease

IBD

◆ Chronic diarrhoea with blood and mucus, and lower-abdominal pain
◆ Fever, mouth ulcers, anorectal disease and extra-intestinal features may be present
◆ Consider in younger patients with above symptoms

Angiodysplasia

◆ Painless bleeding due to enlarged friable blood vessels in colon
◆ Can be bright red, dark blood mixed in with faeces or even present as melaena
◆ Usually occurs in elderly patients

Upper-GI bleed

◆ Dark, tarry stool produced (melaena)
◆ Haematemesis and other alarm symptoms may be present
◆ Previous history of peptic ulcers, chronic liver disease and/or long-term anti-inflammatory use

Investigations

◆ Full abdominal examination, including PR examination and proctoscopy
◆ Bloods – FBC, U&Es, LFT, clotting, CRP, ESR and group and save 2–4 units
◆ Stool culture
◆ Erect chest X-ray – free air under diaphragm indicates perforation
◆ Abdominal X-ray
◆ Sigmoidoscopy/colonoscopy and upper -GIT endoscopy
◆ CT abdomen/pelvis

Management

- Give advice on diet and lifestyle to help with constipation
- Laxatives for constipation exacerbating anorectal and diverticular disease
- Anal fissure – measures to avoid constipation; short course of topical local anaesthetic or steroid cream; GTN ointment and/or surgery in chronic cases
- Haemorrhoids – measures to avoid constipation; rubber-band ligation; sclerosant therapy; haemorrhoidectomy
- Angiodysplasia – ensure patient is haemodynamically stable first; endoscopic obliteration; surgical resection in isolated refractive cases
- 2-week referral for patients with red-flag symptoms
- IBD – stop smoking (Crohn's); sulfasalazine (ulcerative colitis); infliximab in severe disease; surgery; steroids for flare-ups
- Gastroenteritis – rehydration; if history of foreign travel or bloody diarrhoea, consider antibiotics
- Diverticular disease – high-fibre diet and bulk-producing laxatives if no better

Renal medicine & urology

Haematuria 88
Dysuria 92
Polyuria 96

Haematuria

PC
+ Frank haematuria (this history focuses on this presenting complaint)
+ Microscopic haematuria seen on dipstick

HPC
CLOTS
+ **CLarify** – When do you notice the blood? Is it only when you pass urine? Is there any chance it could be coming from elsewhere? What colour is it? Have you recently eaten any beetroot?
+ **Onset** – When did you first notice the blood?
+ **Timing** – Is there always blood in your urine or does it come and go? Have you had this before? Is the blood present at the start of urination, the end or throughout?
+ **Severity** – Do you pass any clots?

Associated symptoms
+ **Pain** – Do you have any pain when you pass urine? Any pain in your tummy or back? *If so, SOCRATES*
+ **Frequency** – Any change in frequency? Any trouble with incontinence? Do you get sudden irrepressible urges to pass water?
+ **Nocturia** – How often do you get up at night to pass urine?
+ **Urinary stream** – Do you have difficulty getting the stream started? Is there prolonged dribbling at the end? Is your stream powerful or weak?
+ **Constitutional** – Have you been unwell recently, or had any fever or chills? How is your appetite? Have you lost any weight?
+ **Renal failure** – Have you gained weight recently? Have your ankles swollen?
+ **Glomerulonephritides** – Have you recently had a sore throat? Have you noticed any rashes or sore joints?
+ **Pulmonary-renal conditions** – Have you recently coughed up any blood?
+ **Trauma** – Have you had any trauma to your stomach or groin recently?

ICE
+ What do you think could be wrong? I know this can be quite a scary problem, but does anything particularly concern you that you would like dealt with?

PMH
+ Do you suffer from any medical conditions?
+ *Ask specifically about previous UTIs, prostate/renal/bladder cancer, BPH, diabetes and hypertension*
+ Have you had a catheter put in recently?

DH
+ Do you take any regular medications?
+ Do you have any allergies?

FH
+ Do any conditions run in the family?
+ *Ask specifically about renal disease (including polycystic kidney disease), bleeding disorders*
+ Does anyone else in the family have blood in their urine? *Asymptomatic haematuria can be benign and familial*

SH
+ Do you smoke? How many do you smoke a day? For how long have you smoked?
+ What is/was your job? Have you ever worked with industrial chemicals or dyes?

Important points
+ Patients may not think that their pink urine contains blood – if they deny blood in their urine, be sure to ask about its colour
+ Presence of clots makes a glomerular cause highly unlikely
+ Timing of haematuria during the urinary stream (i.e. initial, terminal or total) helps to localise the pathology
+ A poor urinary stream suggests there could be an obstructive cause

Differential diagnosis
Haematuria can be gross or microscopic. The causes of these are generally quite different. Gross haematuria is more likely due to a lower-urinary tract lesion, whereas microscopic haematuria is suggestive of glomerular disease. This is not a perfect rule, however. Gross haematuria has a 20%–25% chance of being due to malignancy, which is why it is much more aggressively investigated than microscopic haematuria. Microscopic haematuria is relatively more common, and should only be considered pathological when recurring or associated with lower-urinary tract symptoms.

Malignancy
Renal cell carcinoma
+ Triad of flank pain, haematuria and an abdominal mass (late presentation)
+ Commonly found incidentally in patients with hypertension or anaemia
+ Constitutional symptoms of weight loss, fever and fatigue
+ May present with paraneoplastic syndrome causing excessive renin, parathyroid hormone or erythropoietin

Transitional cell carcinoma
+ Painless, intermittent haematuria in older males is a worrying sign
+ Can affect the ureters or urethra, but most commonly affects the bladder
+ The classical association is working with industrial dyes, but nowadays smoking is by far the biggest risk factor in the UK
+ Schistosomiasis is the biggest cause of bladder cancer elsewhere (e.g. Africa)

Renal calculi

+ Classical presentation – acute onset of excruciating flank/abdominal pain, radiating from 'loin to groin', with associated nausea and vomiting
+ Pain in renal colic is more constant than in biliary/intestinal colic, but often there are periods of relief in which the patient has a dull ache
+ Most often, however, asymptomatic and found incidentally
+ Typically affects men in their thirties to fifties

Urinary tract infection

+ Cystitis typically produces urinary frequency, urgency and dysuria
+ Fever, suprapubic pain and urethral discharge may also be present
+ The urine may be cloudy with a foul odour and of course may contain blood
+ More common in women; in the elderly, the only symptom may be delirium

Glomerulonephritis

+ Can cause nephritis with frank haematuria, or nephrotic syndrome
+ Many different causes; there may be an associated preceding URTI (post-streptococcal or IgA nephropathy); haemoptysis (Goodpasture's syndrome); or systemic features, such as a rash, suggestive of vasculitis

Other

+ Urinary tract injury – blunt, penetrating or iatrogenic (e.g. catheterisation)
+ Coagulopathy, e.g. haemophilia
+ Prostatitis
+ BPH and prostatic carcinoma (although haematuria not typically seen)
+ Beetroot – turns urine pink

Investigations

+ Urinalysis; culture, microscopy and sensitivity to look for UTIs
+ U&Es, FBC and clotting
+ eGFR
+ Autoantibody screen – ANCA, ANA and anti-glomerular basement membrane
+ Urine cytology and cystoscopy for bladder cancer
+ USS renal tract to look for masses
+ Abdominal X-ray
+ IV urography or CT scan if still no cause found
+ Renal biopsy to confirm glomerulonephritis

Management

+ Frank haematuria requires urgent referral on to urology or nephrology
+ Bladder cancer – transurethral resection for superficial tumours; radical cystectomy and urinary diversion for invasive disease; possibly chemotherapy
+ Renal cell carcinoma – nephrectomy
+ Renal calculi – those < 5 mm usually pass on their own; extracorporeal

lithotripsy or endoscopic stone removal for medium-sized stones; rarely, intracorporeal or open operations are required for larger/persistent stones

◆ UTI – antibiotics, e.g. trimethoprim in simple uncomplicated cystitis

◆ Nephrotic syndrome – treat cause; furosemide, ACE inhibitors and calcium channel blockers to control fluid retention and hypertension

◆ Rapidly progressive glomerulonephritis requires prompt treatment with high-dose steroids and cyclophosphamide

Dysuria

HPC

O'SOCRATES

- **Open question** – Can you tell me more about this pain?
- **Site** – Where exactly does it hurt when you pass water? Is it deeper inside or on your skin or genitals?
- **Onset** – When did you first notice the pain?
- **Character** – How would you describe the pain? Burning? Sharp?
- **Radiation** – Does the pain go anywhere else?
- **Associated features** – *see below*
- **Timing** – Is the pain there at the start, towards the end or after passing water? Have you had this pain before?
- **Exacerbating/relieving factors** – Does anything make it better or worse?
- **Severity** – How bad is the pain on a scale of 1–10, with 10 being the worst pain you can imagine?

Urinary history

- **Frequency** – Are you going to the toilet more frequently? Do you pass large or small volumes of urine?
- **Urgency** – Do you get sudden irrepressible urges to pass water?
- **Colour/blood** – Has your urine changed colour? Has there been any blood?
- **Discharge** – Any discharge from your vagina/penis? *If so*, what colour is it? Is it smelly? How long have you had it for? *Take sexual history* (*see* Vaginal discharge, p. 163)
- **Fever** – Have you been feeling unwell? Any fever or shivering?

Urological history (men)

- **Urinary stream** – Do you have difficulty getting the stream started? Is there prolonged dribbling at the end? Is your stream powerful or weak?
- **Nocturia** – How often do you get up at night to pass urine?
- **Prostatitis** – Do you find ejaculation painful?

Gynaecological history (women)

- **Menopause** – Have you gone through the change?
- **Dysmenorrhoea** – Is the pain worse during your periods? Does it stop after you have a period?

Abdominal history

- **Abdo pain** – Do you get pain anywhere in your tummy, sides or in your back other than when you go to the toilet? *If so, SOCRATES*
- **Calculi** – Have you ever passed any stones?
- **Painful motions** – Is it painful to pass bowel motions?
- **Diarrhoea** – In the last month, have you had diarrhoea? Was it bloody?

ICE

- What do you think could be wrong? Does anything particularly concern you that you would like dealt with?

PMH

- Do you suffer from any medical conditions?
- *Ask specifically about previous UTIs, STIs, renal calculi, renal tract injury, arthritis and conjunctivitis*
- Have you had a catheter placed recently?

DH

- Do you take any medications?
- Do you have any allergies?

FH

- Do any conditions run in the family?
- *Ask specifically about any conditions affecting the renal tract, particularly congenital abnormalities that may predispose to UTIs and calculi*

SH

- Does your partner have any similar symptoms?
- Do you smoke? Do you drink alcohol? How much?
- What is your occupation?

Important points

- Important to tailor this history to the individual, e.g. in a 20-year-old female, it may not be important to ask about menopause, but taking a sexual history could elucidate key symptoms
- Pain at the start of urination suggests urethritis, but post-voiding, suprapubic pain is suggestive of cystitis

Differential diagnosis

Urinary tract infection

- Cystitis typically produces urinary frequency, urgency and dysuria
- Fever, suprapubic pain and urethral discharge may also be present
- The urine may be cloudy with a foul odour and may contain blood
- More common in women; in the elderly, the only symptom may be delirium

Pyelonephritis

- Very unwell – fever, rigors, nausea, vomiting, flank pain radiating to the back
- Dysuria, frequency, urgency, nocturia and haematuria may be present

Sexually transmitted infection

- Vaginal/urethral discharge, commonly in young sexually active patients
- Possible history of recent exposure, such as a new partner or unprotected sex
- Possible history of dyspareunia, painful ejaculation or dyschezia (prostatitis)

◆ Reiter's syndrome (reactive arthritis) – urethritis, conjunctivitis and arthritis secondary to STI or gastroenteritis; typically an oligoarthritis

Endometriosis
◆ Cyclical pelvic pain that crescendoes before menstruation and then dissipates
◆ Dyspareunia (deep), dysmenorrhoea, dyschezia, dysuria, subfertility and lower abdominal pain

Atrophic vaginitis
◆ Amenorrhoea, poor tissue elasticity and vaginal dryness and pain
◆ Common in women after menopause and can cause dysuria

Renal calculi
◆ Classical presentation – acute onset of excruciating flank/abdominal pain, radiating from 'loin to groin', with associated nausea and vomiting
◆ Pain in renal colic is more constant than in biliary/intestinal colic, but often has periods of relief in which the patient has a dull ache
◆ Most often, however, asymptomatic and found incidentally
◆ Dysuria may be present due to urinary tract damage
◆ Typically affects men between 30 and 50 years old

Benign prostatic hyperplasia
◆ Urinary frequency and nocturia with obstructive symptoms of hesitancy, terminal dribbling and a weak stream
◆ Incomplete bladder emptying causes continuous urge to go
◆ Haematuria may occur; dysuria occurs due to UTI, secondary to urinary stasis

Investigations
◆ Abdominal examination
◆ PR examination for older men; consider pelvic examination in women
◆ Bloods – FBC, U&Es, CRP and PSA (older men)
◆ Blood cultures where pyelonephritis is suspected
◆ Urine analysis
◆ MSU – culture and sensitivity for UTIs/pyelonephritis
◆ Urethral, high vaginal and endocervical swabs and urine PCR for STIs
◆ Abdominal USS to detect masses
◆ KUB X-ray if suspecting calculi
◆ IV pyelography
◆ Voiding cystourethrography

Management
◆ UTI – antibiotics, e.g. trimethoprim in simple uncomplicated cystitis
◆ Pyelonephritis – antibiotics, e.g. ciprofloxacin; consider admission
◆ STIs – refer to genitourinary medicine; chlamydia and gonorrhoea are best treated with a one-off dose of 1 g azithromycin IM and 500 mg ceftriaxone, respectively; contact tracing should be implemented

◆ Renal calculi – those < 5 mm usually pass on their own; extracorporeal lithotripsy or endoscopic stone removal for medium-sized stones; rarely, intracorporeal or open operations are required for larger/persistent stones
◆ BPH – alpha blockers (e.g. tamsulosin) and 5-alpha reductase inhibitors (e.g. finasteride); transurethral resection of the prostate if medical treatment fails
◆ Atrophic vaginitis – topical lubricants; topical oestrogens or pessaries

Polyuria
HPC
Urinary history
+ **Onset** – When did you start to notice this?
+ **Frequency** – How many times do you pass urine a day? More than six times?
+ **Nocturia** – How often do you get up at night to pass urine? More than twice?
+ **Amount** – How much do you pass each time? Is it large or small amounts?
+ **Thirst** – Are you thirsty? How much fluid do you drink in a day?
+ **Dysuria** – Does it hurt or burn to pass urine?
+ **Haematuria/discharge** – Have you noticed any change in the colour of your urine? Is there any blood or discharge? *If so*, can you describe it please?
+ **Urge incontinence** – Do you ever get a sudden irrepressible urge to pass water? Are you able to hold it in when this happens?

Urological history (men)
+ **Urinary stream** – Do you have difficulty getting the stream started? Is there prolonged dribbling at the end? Is your stream powerful or weak?
+ **Prostatitis** – Do you find ejaculation painful? Any pain passing stool?

Gynaecological history (women)
+ **Prolapse** – Do you have a feeling of fullness or a dropping sensation from your pelvis? Does anything protrude from your vagina, for example when you open your bowels or strain?
+ **Obstetric history** – How many children have you had? Were the births uncomplicated? Were they large babies?
+ **Menopause** – Have you gone through the change yet?

Endocrinological history
+ **Abdo pain** – Have you had any pain in your tummy? *If so, SOCRATES*
+ **Constitutional** – Have you had any recent weight loss? How is your appetite? Have you had a fever recently? Chills?

ICE
+ What do you think could be wrong? Does anything particularly concern you that you would like dealt with?

PMH
+ Do you suffer from any medical conditions?
+ *Ask specifically about diabetes*

DH
+ Do you take any regular medication?
+ *Ask specifically about diuretics*
+ Do you have any allergies?

FH
- Do any conditions run in your family?
- *Ask specifically about diabetes and renal conditions generally*

SH
- Do you smoke? Drink alcohol? How much?
- Are you currently working?

Important points
- Polyuria is defined objectively as the production of more than 3 L of urine in 24 hours, although in practice, finding out the exact volume of urine they are passing from the history is often not possible – it may be necessary to get a voiding diary detailing frequency and volumes of urination
- Again, tailor the history to the patient sat in front of you – in a young woman, the gynaecological history may not be as important as it is in elderly patients, and it may not be appropriate to ask about menopause in such patients

Differential diagnosis
Urinary tract infection
- Cystitis typically produces urinary frequency, urgency and dysuria
- Fever, suprapubic pain and urethral discharge may also be present
- The urine may be cloudy with a foul odour and may contain blood
- More common in women; in the elderly, the only symptom may be delirium

Hyperactive bladder
- Severe urgency, nocturia, frequency and possibly incontinence
- There may be a past history of neurological conditions, such as Parkinson's, stroke or spinal cord disease

Genitourinary prolapse
- Common among older women
- Risk factors include multiple vaginal deliveries, menopause, obesity, complicated vaginal deliveries and hysterectomy
- Symptoms include urinary frequency, recurrent UTIs, stress or urge incontinence and a fullness sensation in the vagina

Benign prostatic hyperplasia
- Urinary frequency and nocturia with obstructive symptoms of hesitancy, terminal dribbling and a weak stream
- Incomplete bladder emptying causes continuous urge to go
- Haematuria and dysuria may also occur

Diabetes mellitus
- Polydipsia and polyuria, with abdominal pain, nausea, vomiting, weight loss and 'pear drop' breath seen in diabetic ketoacidosis
- May be presenting feature, particularly in type 1 diabetes mellitus

◆ Often a family history of diabetes

Diabetes insipidus
◆ Polydipsia and polyuria
◆ Patients produce huge quantities of very dilute urine (almost pure water); they are rarely dehydrated unless prevented from drinking large quantities of water
◆ Nocturia is often present and bothersome; however, there are no symptoms suggestive of an obstructive or irritative urinary disorder
◆ Can be inherited, presenting within the first few years of life

Others
◆ Iatrogenic – diuretics used to treat hypertension are a very common cause
◆ Psychogenic polydipsia – patient drinks beyond true water requirement; more common nowadays due to belief that drinking lots of water is healthy
◆ Hypercalcaemia – abdominal pain, vomiting, drowsiness, confusion, anorexia, muscle weakness and constipation; malignancy, Paget's disease of bone and hyperparathyroidism are all recognised causes
◆ Hypokalaemia – non-specific symptoms of constipation, weakness and confusion; augmented by diarrhoea, vomiting, diuretics and laxative abuse

Investigations
◆ Abdominal examination
◆ PR examination for older men; consider pelvic examination in women
◆ FBC, U&Es, fasting glucose and PSA (older men)
◆ Urine osmolality to see if it is a solute or water diuresis
◆ Urine analysis
◆ MSU sample – culture and sensitivity
◆ Urodynamic investigation
◆ Water-deprivation test

Management
◆ UTI – antibiotics, e.g. trimethoprim in simple uncomplicated cystitis
◆ Diabetes mellitus – insulin regime for type 1 diabetics; diet-controlled or treated with metformin (and possibly hypoglycaemics) for type 2 diabetics
◆ In diabetic ketoacidosis, emergency admission with fluid and electrolyte resuscitation is required initially, with insulin until glucose level is controlled
◆ Diabetes insipidus – careful regular fluid intake may suffice in mild cases; exogenous antidiuretic hormone is given where this is not sufficient
◆ Genitourinary prolapse – *Vaginal pessaries*; surgery to tighten and reattach the pelvic ligaments in younger patients or where pessaries aren't sufficient
◆ BPH – alpha blockers (e.g. tamsulosin) and 5-alpha reductase inhibitors (e.g. finasteride); transurethral resection of the prostate if medical treatment fails
◆ Hyperactive bladder – pelvic floor exercises; cutting out caffeine and alcohol; anticholinergics (e.g. oxybutynin); surgery, e.g. sacral nerve stimulation or intravesical botulinum toxin may be considered in refractory cases
◆ Diuretics (iatrogenic) – take once in the morning to avoid disturbed nights

- Hypercalcaemia – treat cause; fluids; bisphosphonates; loop diuretics
- Hypokalaemia – treat cause; the severity of the deficit and clinical findings dictate whether intensive replacement or conservative measures are necessary

Neurology

Falls 102
Headache 106
Weakness 110
Numbness/paraesthesia 114
Dizziness 118
Hearing loss 121

Falls

HPC

Before

- **Open question** – Can you talk me through what happened exactly? Where and when? What were you doing at the time?
- **Aura** – How did you feel immediately before the episode? Any aura? Chest pain, anxious or fearful? Did you have any warning that something was about to happen?
- **Environmental** – Did you trip over anything or slip?
- **LOC** – Did you lose consciousness? How long for?
- **Witness** – Did anyone witness the episode? How did they describe the episode?

During

- **Fall** – How did you fall exactly? Did you hit your head?
- **Seizure** – Did you have a fit? Can you describe it? Did your whole body shake or only part of it?
- **Continence** – Did you pass any urine or soil yourself?
- **Tongue** – Did you bite your tongue? *If yes*, was it the front or the side?

After

- **Post-ictal state** – How did you feel immediately after the fall/when you regained consciousness? Were you confused? Drowsy? Aching muscles?
- **Todd's paralysis** – Did you have any weakness afterwards?
- **Previous episodes** – Has something like this ever happened before? *If yes*, can you describe exactly what happened those times?
- **Eyesight** – How is your eyesight? Do you have difficulty getting about?
- **Cardio** – Do you suffer from chest pain at all? Do you get breathless often?

ICE

- What do you think is wrong? Is there anything you are particularly worried about or would like to discuss?

PMH

- Do you suffer from any medical conditions?
- *Ask specifically about epilepsy, hypertension and arrhythmias*

DH

- Are you taking any medications? Have any been changed or added recently?
- *Ask specifically about blood pressure drugs, sedatives and antidepressants*
- Allergies?

FH

- Do any conditions run in your family?
- *Ask specifically about epilepsy and arrhythmias*

SH

+ How much alcohol do you drink? Had you been drinking at the time of your fall?
+ Do you smoke? How many do/did you smoke? How many years have you smoked/did you smoke for?
+ Do you take any recreational drugs?
+ Are you in work/employed? What effect has this had on your job?
+ *If it could be a fit, ask them about driving*
+ What effect have these fall(s) had on your life?
+ Who is at home? Do you have stairs? Have you had any modifications put in place, such as rails or a chairlift?

Important points

+ It is important to verify if anyone else witnessed the episode and make it clear that you would like to get their story of events
+ A detailed description of the episode is crucial – subtle differences will help distinguish a true epileptic seizure from syncopal episodes
+ Always consider the damage the fall has done as well – did they hit their head and is there any indication of trauma elsewhere?

Differential diagnosis

The aetiology of a fall is often multifactorial, particularly in elderly patients. Vasovagal syncope is very common, as is postural hypotension in older individuals who are often on medication for hypertension. It is important not to forget as well that many older individuals are frail, with poor eyesight, and simple measures should be taken to help prevent falls, e.g. ensuring their home environment is safe and suitable for them.

Seizure

+ Can be partial or generalised (involving both hemispheres); simple or complex (impaired consciousness)
+ Sequence of events (generalised tonic–clonic):
  + Patient loses consciousness → falls → limbs go stiff → limbs jerk violently (10–20 seconds)
  + Aura may precede episode (visual, olfactory, sensory, déjà vu)
  + Biting side of tongue and urinary/faecal incontinence are features
  + A post-ictal state of drowsiness, myalgia, headache and amnesia is common
  + Can last up to 2–3 minutes

Vasovagal syncope

+ Evoked by strong emotion (e.g. fear), pain or prolonged standing
+ Nausea, pallor and sweating often precede episode by a few seconds
+ Brief loss of consciousness, lasting no more than 2 minutes generally
+ Limb jerking is uncommon, but may occur (no tonic–clonic sequence)
+ No post-ictal state

Postural hypotension
+ Patient moves from lying/sitting position to standing
+ Very brief episode (lasting a few seconds)
+ 'Head rush' or unsteadiness
+ Tricyclic antidepressants or antihypertensive meds may contribute

Carotid sinus syncope
+ Turning of the head or shaving can lead to brief loss of consciousness

Situational syncope
+ Micturition (particularly men at night) or a coughing attack may precipitate syncope

Stokes–Adams attack
+ Patient falls to ground, appearing pale, with a slow or absent pulse
+ Rapid recovery, with pulse returning to normal and facial flushing

Aortic stenosis
+ Central chest pain and shortness of breath on effort
+ Older patients generally (senile calcification of aortic valve)

Myocardial infarction
+ Crushing central chest pain that may radiate to an arm and/or jaw
+ Nausea, sweating and dyspnoea
+ In older patients, may present simply as syncope, without chest pain

Poor eyesight and/or mobility
+ Older individuals with arthritis, poor eyesight and/or poor balance are at greater risk of falling
+ May trip over loose carpets, wires, objects on floor, etc.

Investigations
+ Full cardiovascular and neurological examination
+ Assess gait, balance, vision, cognition and risk of osteoporosis
+ Bloods – FBC and U&Es
+ ECG – myocardial infarction and arrhythmias
+ 24-Hour ECG – transient arrhythmia, e.g. Stokes–Adams attack
+ Lying and standing blood pressure – drop of > 20/10 mmHg = postural hypotension
+ Echocardiogram – aortic stenosis; hypertrophic obstructive cardiomyopathy in young

Management
+ Avoid precipitating factors (e.g. tell patients to get up slowly and carefully, not suddenly)
+ Involve social workers and occupational therapists

◆ Ensure the patient's home environment is safe – consider rails, chairlifts or even moving to sheltered accommodation
◆ Review medication – do they need to be on all their tablets?
◆ Strength and balance training
◆ If recurrent seizures, educate and consider therapy
◆ Treat myocardial infarction and aortic stenosis appropriately

Headache
HPC
O'SOCRATES
- **Open question** – Would you please tell me about your headaches?
- **Site** – *ask about frontal, occipital, temporal, unilateral, all over*
- **Onset** – Did it come on suddenly? Do you have any warnings prior to the headache?
- **Character** – Was it one episode or multiple? Describe the pain
- **Radiation** – Does the pain move anywhere else?
- **Associated symptoms** – *see below*
- **Timing** – When can you remember this starting? Was it continuous or intermittent? How long do they last? When was the last time you had a headache?
- **Exacerbating or relieving factors** – Does it get worse on coughing? Is it worse at night or in the early morning? Any particular activities or movements? Does anything relieve the pain?
- **Severity** – How bad is the pain on a scale of 1–10, with 10 being the worst pain you can imagine? Has it changed over time? How is it now? Is it painful to touch or press over?

Associated features
- **Fever** – Have you been feeling ill or had a fever?
- **Trauma** – Have you banged your head, had a fall recently?
- **Sensorimotor changes** – Have you had any arm or leg weakness? Any visual disturbances? Any other sensory disturbance? Have you ever lost consciousness?
- **Meningism** – Are you sensitive to light? Do you have any neck stiffness? Have you noticed a rash anywhere?
- **Seizures/blackouts** – Have you ever had seizures or blacked out?
- **Sentinel headache** – *If acute*, have you had a less severe headache recently?
- **Inflammatory** – Is it painful to comb your hair or to chew? Do you have any visual changes? Do you have any pain or aches in your shoulders?
- **Vision** – Any eye pain? Visual disturbances? Nausea or vomiting?

ICE
- Have you got any idea what is causing the headache? What concerns you most about this headache? How does it affect your day-to-day living? How badly do you want something done about it?

PMH
- Do you suffer from any other medical conditions?
- *Ask specifically about migraines, polycystic kidney disease and polymyalgia rheumatica (if suspecting temporal arteritis)*
- Have you ever had something like this before?
- Have you travelled abroad recently?

DH

+ Are you taking any medications? Have any of these been changed or added recently?
+ Do you have any allergies?

FH

+ Do any conditions run in your family?
+ *Ask specifically about bleeding disorders and polycystic kidney disease*

SH

+ How much alcohol do you drink?
+ Do you smoke? How many do/did you smoke? For how many years?
+ Do you take any recreational drugs?
+ Are you in work? What effect has this had on your job?
+ Who is at home? How does this affect you at home? Have you had any modifications put in place?

Important points

+ After asking open questions, it is best to characterise it first into whether it is unilateral or bilateral, the kind of pain involved and associated symptoms to gain a quick idea of which line of questioning to take
+ It is important to exclude potential life-threatening causes by asking about red-flag symptoms
+ Never forget to consider emergencies, such as subarachnoid or extradural haemorrhage, meningitis, temporal arteritis, angle-closure glaucoma, raised intracranial pressure (e.g. due to tumour or venous sinus thrombosis) and subdural haemorrhage. These can be more easily memorised by starting in the brain parenchyma (tumour), then the vessels (haemorrhage and clots), then the meninges (meningitis), then extracranial arteries (temporal arteritis) and finally the eye (glaucoma)

Differential diagnosis

When considering the working diagnosis, one of the first questions you should consider is whether the headache is recurring or happening for the first time. Headaches occurring for the first time obviously could still be migraine, cluster headaches or tension headaches, but it is important to try to rule out sinister causes.

Migraine

+ Severe, pulsating, recurring, unilateral headache that lasts around an hour
+ Often has visual or sensory 'aura', occurring shortly before onset
+ Photophobia/phonophobia when headache starts, patient seeks dark quiet room
+ Triggers – changes in diet, oral contraceptives, exercise, caffeine and alcohol

Cluster headache

+ Excruciating, recurring, unilateral headache normally localised around one eye
+ Lasts for only a few hours, often twice in 24 hours and most common at night
+ Headaches occur in clusters for weeks, then headache-free for months
+ Associated with profuse eye watering and nasal secretions on the affected side

Tension headache

+ Bilateral and associated with stress and visual strain (reading, watching TV)
+ Typically described as a tight band across the head that lasts minutes–hours
+ No other signs or symptoms

Sinusitis

+ Pain over sinuses (e.g. behind eyes or deep behind nose)
+ Constant dull ache, associated with coryzal symptoms, fever and congestion
+ Worse on bending forwards

Meningitis

+ Classical presentation – headache, fever, neck stiffness and photophobia
+ Non-blanching purpuric rash indicates meningococcal septicaemia
+ Later presentation includes seizures, decreased conscious level and even coma

Extradural haemorrhage

+ Typically due to trauma to the temple, damaging the middle meningeal artery
+ There may be a lucid interval, with increasingly severe headache, associated raised ICP symptoms and gradually decreasing consciousness until complete loss

Subdural haemorrhage

+ Common in elderly after falling/banging their head in previous weeks/months
+ Worsening pain, decreasing consciousness, increased sleepiness and ataxia
+ ICP gradually increases until it causes symptoms (*see below*)

Subarachnoid haemorrhage

+ Sudden, severe 'thunderclap' headache, sometimes with a sentinel headache of less severity within the weeks prior to the current headache
+ Linked to polycystic kidney disease, and Ehlers–Danlos syndrome

Raised intracranial pressure

+ Often described as 'worst headache ever'
+ Morning headache, worse on coughing, lying down or any Valsalva manoeuvre
+ May have visual disturbances, seizures and other neurological symptoms

Temporal arteritis
- Severe headache located in the temple area
- Jaw claudication, scalp tenderness; often polymyalgia rheumatic symptoms
- Sudden blindness in one eye if not treated promptly

Others
- Angle-closure glaucoma – acute painful red eye, visual halos, reduced vision
- Medication – mixed analgesics may cause a headache themselves
- Trigeminal neuralgia – short, intense 'electric shock' pain in trigeminal nerve distribution triggered by touching affected area (e.g. shaving or brushing hair)

Investigations
- Neurological examination and examination for tender areas over skull
- Ophthalmoscopy (for evidence of papilloedema)
- Bloods – FBC, U&Es, CRP and ESR
- Temporal artery biopsy if temporal arteritis suspected
- CT/MRI scan
- Lumbar puncture if not contraindicated

Management
- General – analgesia and hydration; ABCDE approach if acutely unwell
- Migraine – avoid precipitants; triptan (e.g. sumatriptan) when headache starts
- Cluster headache – 100% oxygen and sumatriptan for acute attacks; verapamil or prednisolone for prophylaxis
- Meningitis – IV antibiotics (e.g. cefotaxime)
- Intracranial haemorrhage – neurosurgery (e.g. craniotomy plus evacuation)
- Raised ICP – elevate head of bed to 30 degrees; sedation, cerebrospinal fluid drainage, mannitol, neuromuscular blockade and hyperventilation lower ICP
- Temporal arteritis – high-dose oral prednisolone

Weakness
HPC
O'SOCRATES
+ **Open question** – Can you tell me exactly what you have noticed?
+ **Site** – Where is the weakness? Legs? Arms? Facial muscles? One side or both?
+ **Onset** – When did you first notice it? Did it come on suddenly or gradually? *If suddenly*, what were you doing at the time?
+ **Character** – Is the weakness always there or does it vary significantly?
+ **Radiation** – Do you have weakness anywhere else?
+ **Associated features** – *see later*
+ **Timing** – How has it changed over time? Has it ever happened before?
+ **Exacerbating/relieving factors** – Does anything make it worse or better? Does it change with heat? Do your muscles tire easily?
+ **Severity** – How bad is the weakness? Do you have any movement? Are you able to walk/use your arms? Where is it worst?

Associated features
+ **Sensory** – Any numbness or tingling anywhere? Have you noticed any changes in your vision? Hearing? Taste? Smell?
+ **Muscle wasting** – Have you noticed a reduction in muscle bulk in the areas affected?
+ **Balance** – Any problems with your balance?
+ **Speech** – Have you had any trouble with your speech previously?
+ **Headaches** – Have you had any bad headaches recently? *If so, SOCRATES*
+ **Seizures and blackouts** – Have you had any seizures or blackouts?
+ **Pain** – Have you had any back pain or pain elsewhere? *If so, SOCRATES*
+ **Incontinence** – Have you had any trouble with your waterworks or bowels? Do you suffer from incontinence of urine or stools? (*Ask sensitively!*)
+ **Constitutional** – Have you felt ill or feverish recently? Have you noticed any weight loss? How has your appetite been? Have you been feeling tired?

ICE
+ What do you think is wrong? Is there anything you are particularly worried about or would like to discuss? How does this affect you day to day?

PMH
+ Do you suffer from any medical conditions?
+ *Ask specifically about diabetes and spinal pathology*

DH
+ Are you taking any medications? Have any of these been changed or added recently?
+ *Ask specifically about long-term corticosteroids*
+ Do you have any allergies?

FH
◆ Do any conditions run in your family?
◆ *Ask specifically about muscular dystrophy and autoimmune disorders*

SH
◆ Do you drink alcohol? How much do you drink in a week?
◆ Do you smoke? How many do/did you smoke? For how many years?
◆ Do you take any recreational drugs?
◆ Are you in work/employed? What effect has this had on your job?
◆ Who is at home? How does this affect you at home? Have you had any modifications put in place?

Important points
◆ It is important to clarify exactly which parts of the body are affected by the weakness – upper/lower limbs, left/right, proximal/distal muscles, as this will help aid diagnosis
◆ During the history, you should be trying to localise where the problem lies – does it lie in the muscles, neuromuscular junction, peripheral nerve, plexus, nerve root, spinal cord or the brain?
◆ The nature of the weakness will provide many clues – muscles that quickly fatigue and lose power may indicate myasthenia gravis, whereas an acute onset of muscle weakness affecting only one side is typical of a stroke

Differential diagnosis
There are seven broad areas that can cause symptoms of weakness. If you split your history taking up with these in mind, it may help: muscle, neuromuscular junction, peripheral nerve, plexus, nerve root, spinal cord and the brain.

Muscles
Muscular dystrophy (e.g. Duchenne's and Becker's muscular dystrophy)
◆ Onset usually during childhood
◆ Painless gradual weakness predominantly affecting proximal limb muscles
◆ Difficultly standing up/walking

Polymyositis/dermatomyositis
◆ Slow-onset proximal muscle weakness and myalgia – difficultly standing up/walking
◆ Fever, subcutaneous calcifications, Raynaud's phenomenon and interstitial lung disease may be present
◆ Dermatomyositis involves skin – cracked dry skin on hands, heliotrope rash around eyes, macular rash ('shawl sign' over the shoulders), Gottron's papules over knuckles

Muscle wasting from disuse
◆ Patients who are bedridden for a period of time
◆ Patients who have had a limb cast

Neuromuscular junction
Myasthenia gravis
+ Autoimmune condition in which patient's muscles become weak after use
+ Often affects face, eye movement and eyelid muscles most
+ Also causes a proximal myopathy, with symptoms worse at end of the day
+ Thymoma often present

Lambert-Eaton myasthenic syndrome
+ Paraneoplastic syndrome that unlike myasthenia gravis spares the eyes
+ Patient's weakness improves on repeated use of the muscle

Peripheral nerves – *see* Numbness/paraesthesia, p. 116
+ Peripheral neuropathy
+ Mononeuropathy
+ Mononeuritis multiplex

Radiculopathy/plexopathy – *see* Numbness/paraesthesia, pp. 115–16

Spinal cord – *see* Numbness/paraesthesia, p. 116
+ Cervical spondylosis
+ Syringomyelia
+ Spinal stenosis

Central – *see* Numbness/paraesthesia, p. 115
+ Multiple sclerosis
+ Stroke
+ Tumour/abscess

Motor neurone disease
+ Gradual loss of upper and lower motor neurones
+ Limb weakness (e.g. dropping objects and/or 'heavy' legs), speech problems, dysphagia and dyspnoea, but no sensory or sphincter loss
+ Often > 40 years old
+ Difficulties with activities of daily living
+ Rule out other causes of weakness first

Investigations
+ Full neurological examination (lower limb, upper limb and cranial nerves)
+ Bloods – FBC, U&Es, creatine kinase, autoimmune screen
+ Chest X-ray
+ Nerve conduction studies
+ Tensilon test for myasthenia gravis
+ CT/MRI brain/spinal cord/both (depending on clinical findings)

Management

- Encourage physical activity and offer physiotherapy
- Muscular dystrophy – support, genetic counselling; orthoses and prednisolone may help prolong ambulatory phase
- Polymyositis – immunosuppression with oral prednisolone
- Myasthenia gravis – acetylcholinesterase inhibitors, immunosuppression with steroids and/or steroid-sparing agents; thymectomy
- Motor neurone disease – palliative care through a multidisciplinary approach, including physiotherapy, speech and language therapy, occupational therapy and gastrostomy for dysphagia; riluzole may prolong life by around 3 months
- Others – *see* Numbness/paraesthesia, p. 117

Numbness/paraesthesia

HPC

O'SOCRATES

- **Open question** – I understand that you have some odd feelings in (e.g.) your legs. Would you like to tell me about the problem?
- **Site** – Where do you get this feeling? Does it affect both sides of the body?
- **Onset and timing** – When can you remember this starting? Have you always had this? Did it come on suddenly or over some time?
- **Character** – Can you describe what it feels like exactly?
- **Radiation** – Do you have the same odd feelings anywhere else?
- **Associated factors** – Do you have any other symptoms? Do you ever feel anxious before it happens?
- **Timing** – Is it there all the time or does it come and go? How has it changed over time? When is it worst? When is it best? How is it now?
- **Exacerbating/relieving factors** – What, if anything, brings it on? Is it worse with stress? Heat? Exercise?
- **Severity** – How badly is it affecting you day to day?

Associated features

- **Sensory** – Do you have any numbness/tingling (*if not previously mentioned*)? Have you noticed any changes in vision or eye pain? Hearing? Taste? Smell?
- **Motor** – Any feelings of weakness? Any difficulty with daily activities?
- **Balance** – Any problems with your balance?
- **Speech** – Have you had any trouble with your speech previously?
- **Headaches** – Have you had any bad headaches recently? *If so, SOCRATES*
- **Seizures and blackouts** – Have you had any seizures or blackouts?
- **Pain** – Have you had any back pain or pain elsewhere? *If so, SOCRATES*
- **Incontinence** – Have you had any trouble with your waterworks or bowels? Do you suffer from incontinence of urine or stools? (*Ask sensitively!*)
- **Constitutional** – Have you felt ill or feverish recently? Have you noticed any weight loss? How has your appetite been? Have you been feeling tired?

Non-neurological causes

- **Anxiety** – Do you ever feel panicked or anxious each time before it happens?
- **Vascular** – Does it happen when your hands or feet are cold? Do your hands/feet turn white, then blue, then red? Is it painful when they are red?

ICE

- What do you think is wrong? Is there anything you are particularly worried about or would like to discuss? What would you like to be done about this?

PMH

- Do you suffer from any medical conditions?
- *Ask specifically about diabetes, stress and previous surgery*

DH
+ Are you taking any medications? Have any of these been changed or added recently?
+ Do you have any allergies?

FH
+ Do any conditions run in your family?
+ *Ask specifically about diabetes and neurological conditions*

SH
+ Do you drink alcohol? How much do you drink in a week? Is this a typical week? (*Ask CAGE questions if considering alcohol as a cause of neuropathy*)
+ Do you smoke? How many do/did you smoke? For how many years?
+ Do you take any recreational drugs?
+ Are you in work/employed? What effect has this had on your job?

Important points
+ The key to this history is to differentiate between a pathological cause of paraesthesia and a supratentorial cause – this can be difficult
+ Beware the patient who describes numbness 'all over'!
+ During the history, you should be trying to localise where the problem lies – does it lie in the muscles, neuromuscular junction, peripheral nerve, plexus, nerve root, spinal cord or the brain?

Differential diagnosis
Central
Multiple sclerosis
+ Demyelinating disorder diagnosed by clinical, laboratory or radiological evidence of central nervous system lesions disseminated in time and space
+ Common presentations – optic neuritis, altered sensation, weakness and ataxia
+ INSULAR – Intention tremor, Nystagmus, Slurred speech, Urogenital symptoms, Labile emotions, Ataxia, Retrobulbar neuritis

Stroke/transient ischaemic attack
+ Sudden onset, affecting any part(s) of the central nervous system
+ Other neurological symptoms likely, e.g. motor, speech and eyesight problems

Tumour/abscess
+ Slowly evolving symptoms, such as seizures, focal neurological deficits, cognitive/personality changes and signs of raised ICP (*see headache history*)

Spinal cord
Radiculopathy/plexopathy
+ Pressure on nerve root affecting sensory or motor modalities from that root

◆ Meralgia paraesthetica – a common benign complaint of thigh numbness due to irritation of the lateral cutaneous nerve of the thigh
◆ Shingles causes intense pain and blistering in a dermatomal distribution

Cervical spondylosis
◆ Altered sensation below level affected; neck stiffness possible
◆ Upper limbs – LMN signs
◆ Lower limbs – UMN signs

Spinal stenosis
◆ Pressure on spine from mass, trauma or spondylolisthesis
◆ Sensory level with altered sensation below affected level
◆ LMN signs at affected level, with UMN signs below affected level

Syringomyelia
◆ Specific area of sensory or motor loss related to location of syrinx
◆ Usually one sensory tract is lost at a time, e.g. spinothalamic tract
◆ Symptoms may worsen due to events such as trauma, sneezing or coughing

Peripheral neuropathy
Mononeuropathy – e.g. due to trauma, carpal tunnel syndrome or infection
◆ Affects a single dermatome and/or myotome; can be motor, sensory or both
◆ Can happen following trauma/nerve compression, e.g. pressure on the medial epicondyle of the humerus may lead to ulnar nerve palsy
◆ Carpal tunnel syndrome – pain and numbness in median nerve distribution; typically at night, with patient waking and shaking their hand to relieve it

Mononeuritis multiplex – e.g. due to diabetes, autoimmune, infections or amyloidosis
◆ Inflammation of multiple single peripheral nerves, causing pain, numbness and weakness, associated with the above conditions

Polyneuropathy
◆ Causes (ABCDE) – Alcohol, vitamin B deficiency, Chronic renal failure, Diabetes and Everything else (e.g. multiple sclerosis, cancer, amyloidosis)
◆ Can be mainly motor or sensory ('glove and stocking' distribution) or mixed

Non-neurological causes
Anxiety attacks (± hyperventilation)
◆ History of anxiety, with tingling sensations around mouth and in fingers
◆ Sympathetic response – tachycardia, sweating, trembling and/or shaking

Raynaud's phenomenon
◆ Hands turn from white to blue to red (with severe pain), often when cold
◆ Primary Raynaud's is very common and benign; secondary causes include autoimmune conditions, e.g. scleroderma and lupus – distal necrosis/ulcers

Investigations

- ◆ Neurological examination
- ◆ Bloods – FBC, U&Es, vitamin levels, HbA1C (if diabetic), gamma-GT
- ◆ Nerve conduction studies
- ◆ CT/MRI brain/spinal cord/both (depending on clinical findings)

Management

- ◆ Multiple sclerosis – symptomatic treatment (e.g. analgesia); steroids for flare-ups; azathioprine and interferon may be considered to reduce relapses
- ◆ Stroke – early intervention imperative; aspirin initially; thrombolysis in ischaemic stroke; neurosurgery in haemorrhagic stroke
- ◆ Treat underlying cause of peripheral neuropathies, e.g. carpal tunnel syndrome – local steroid injection or carpal tunnel release surgery if problematic

Dizziness

HPC

O'SOCRATES

- **Open question** – Can you tell me more about your dizziness?
- **Specify** – What exactly do you mean when you say you feel 'dizzy'? Does it feel as if the room is spinning around you? *Or,* do you mean you feel like you're going to faint? *Or,* do you feel unsteady on your feet and fall over?
- **Onset** – When did you first notice this? Does it come on suddenly or slowly?
- **Character** – Can you describe exactly how you feel when it comes on?
- **Radiation** – Have you noticed a ringing in your ears?
- **Associated features** – Have you noticed any deafness? Have you felt unwell at all? Any ear pain? Have you felt sick? *If so,* have you been sick at all?
- **Timing** – Is it there all the time or does it come and go? What are you doing when it comes on?
- **Exacerbating/relieving factors** – Does anything bring it on? Does it happen when you try to stand up? *If so,* do you ever get it when you are sitting down? Does anything make it better or worse? Is it made worse when you move or turn your head? Do you feel particularly anxious or worried before it happens?
- **Severity** – Has it ever caused you to have a fall? *If so,* do you find you always fall to the same side?

Neurological symptoms

- **Sensory** – Do you have any numbness/tingling anywhere? Have you noticed any changes in vision or eye pain?
- **Motor** – Any feelings of weakness? Any difficulty with daily activities?
- **Speech** – Have you had any trouble with your speech previously?
- **Headaches** – Have you had any bad headaches recently? *If so, SOCRATES*
- **Seizures and blackouts** – Have you had any seizures or blackouts?
- **Constitutional** – Have you noticed any weight loss? How is your appetite?

ICE

- What do you think is wrong? Is there anything you are particularly worried about or would like to discuss? What would you like to be done about this?

PMH

- Do you suffer from any medical conditions?
- *Ask specifically about previous strokes, recent infections and recent trauma*

DH

- Are you taking any medications? Have any of these been changed recently?
- Do you have any allergies?

FH

- Do any conditions run in the family?
- *Ask specifically about genetic conditions*

SH
+ Do you drink alcohol? If so, how much? Are you under the influence when the dizziness comes on?
+ Do you smoke? How many cigarettes do you smoke a day? For how long have you smoked?
+ Do you take any recreational drugs?
+ Are you in work/employed? What effect has this had on your job?

Important points
+ 'Dizziness' can mean different things to different people – it is important to clarify early on exactly what the patient means by the term
+ Vertigo is the sensation that the patient or the room they are in is spinning, often coupled with nausea and nystagmus
+ In pre-syncope, the patient may be feeling faint or light-headed
+ They may mean they are unsteady on their feet and keep falling over (*see* Falls, p. 102)
+ Feelings of dizziness can also be of psychiatric origin

Differential diagnosis
Benign paroxysmal positional vertigo
+ Usually only lasts for seconds
+ Normally due to moving head
+ No deafness or tinnitus

Acute labyrinthitis
+ Sudden onset
+ Can be severe, with nausea and vomiting
+ Usually no deafness or tinnitus (sudden deafness requires emergency referral)
+ Can be viral or vascular in origin

Ménière's disease
+ Progressive deafness
+ Attacks of vertigo with nausea, tinnitus and a feeling of ear fullness occur in clusters
+ Associated with high-salt diets and alcohol, caffeine and tobacco consumption

Acoustic neuroma
+ Unilateral hearing loss with focal neurological deficits (e.g. facial numbness)
+ Symptoms of raised ICP (e.g. morning headache)
+ Associated with neurofibromatosis type 2

Ototoxicity
+ Streptomycin, vancomycin, gentamicin, chloroquines and chemotherapy are all potentially ototoxic drugs
+ Deafness and tinnitus

Herpes zoster oticus (Ramsay Hunt syndrome)

- Reactivation of latent varicella zoster virus in geniculate ganglion of the facial nerve
- Presenting feature is typically an extremely painful blistered external meatus
- Facial palsy, deafness and tinnitus may also present

Trauma

- Head injury
- Decreased level of consciousness

Other

- Migraine with aura
- Stroke/transient ischaemic attack
- Multiple sclerosis
- Intracranial haemorrhage

Investigations

- Neurological examination, including cranial nerves and gait assessment
- Eye examination for nystagmus
- Otoscopy
- Dix–Hallpike test for BPPV
- Bloods – FBC, U&Es, LFTs, glucose and CRP
- Pure-tone audiometry
- Allergy testing
- Electronystagmography
- ECG
- CT/MRI head

Management

- General – review medication and stop ototoxic drugs; consider risk towards driving and occupational hazards; treat vertigo and nausea acutely with anti-emetics (e.g. prochlorperazine) and consider vestibular rehabilitation programmes – may help long term
- BPPV – Epley manoeuvre
- Acute labyrinthitis – bed rest and anti-emetics
- Ménière's disease – diet low in salt and avoiding alcohol, caffeine and tobacco may help prevent attacks; prophylactic betahistine may be of benefit; anti-emetics for acute attacks; hearing aids
- Acoustic neuroma – watchful waiting; if growing, consider surgery and/or radiotherapy
- Herpes zoster oticus – analgesia; acyclovir within 72 hours of the onset of rash

Hearing loss

There are numerous causes of childhood deafness; however, this chapter will deal with those of adult onset.

HPC

O'SOCRATES

+ **Open question** – What exactly have you noticed?
+ **Site** – Is one ear better than the other or are both affected? Which ear did it start in?
+ **Onset** – When did you first notice this? Did it come on suddenly or gradually? *If suddenly*, what were you doing at the time? (*Barotrauma – e.g. deep sea diving, sudden explosive noises and head trauma*)
+ **Character** – Do you find any particular noises hard to hear? (*High/low pitched noises*)
+ **Radiation** – Do you get a ringing noise in either ear? *If so*, which did you notice first?
+ **Associated features** – *see later*
+ **Timing** – Have you always been hard of hearing? Has it changed over time?
+ **Exacerbating/relieving factors** – Are there particular times you find it even harder than usual to hear? Does anything make it better or worse? Is it better, worse or the same when there is background noise?
+ **Severity** – How has this affected your day-to-day life?

Associated features

+ **Vertigo** – Do you ever feel as if the room is spinning around you?
+ **Discharge** – Have you had any discharge from either ear? *If so*, what colour is it? Is it smelly?
+ **Foreign bodies** – Do you ever clean your ears with cotton buds or anything else?
+ **Balance** – Any problems with your balance?
+ **Sensory** – Any numbness or tingling anywhere (particularly in the face)?
+ **Motor** – Any feelings of weakness (particularly in the face)?
+ **Headaches** – Have you had any headaches recently? *If so, SOCRATES*
+ **Infection** – Have you felt ill or feverish recently? *Postinfective hearing loss – HIS MMM: Herpes, Influenza, Syphilis, Measles, Mumps, Meningitis*
+ **Weight loss** – Have you noticed any weight loss? How has your appetite been? Have you been feeling tired?

ICE

+ What do you think is wrong? Is there anything you are particularly worried about or would like to discuss?

PMH

+ Do you suffer from any medical conditions?

DH

◆ Are you taking any medications?
◆ *Ask specifically about antibiotics (streptomycin, vancomycin and gentamicin), chloroquines and chemotherapy – 'Voices More Quiet': Vincristine, Mycins, chloroQuine.*
◆ Do you have any allergies?

FH

◆ Do any conditions run in your family?
◆ Any problems with deafness? *If so*, at what age did the family member become deaf? Did they have any other problems (tinnitus, vertigo, other neurology)?

SH

◆ What hobbies do you have? Do you listen to loud music or attend rock concerts?
◆ What do/did you do for a living?
◆ How much alcohol do you drink?
◆ Do you smoke? How many do/did you smoke? For how many years?
◆ Who is at home? How does this affect you at home? Have you had any modifications put in place?

Important points

◆ When speaking to someone who is hard of hearing, it is important to clarify at the beginning of the consultation how easy it will be to communicate
◆ To aid communication, try to find if one ear is better than the other, decrease background noise and sit at the same level so they can see your mouth moving
◆ Try to pick short sentences when asking questions, speak loudly and clearly; you may need to arrange for a sign-language translator to be present
◆ The presence or absence of tinnitus, vertigo, balance and other neurological symptoms will aid diagnosis
◆ The social history can delineate many causes of hearing loss/tinnitus, e.g. attending loud rock concerts, working with pneumatic drills, etc.

Differential diagnosis

Conductive hearing loss

External canal pathology

◆ Wax or foreign bodies such as the tips of cotton buds
◆ Infective causes such as granulation tissue

Tympanic membrane perforation

◆ Often due to rapid pressure changes, such as on a plane, diving, or an explosion; can also be due to infection

Otitis media with effusion

◆ 'Glue ear' is the commonest cause of hearing loss in childhood
◆ Earache may also be present, with fluid accumulation in the middle ear

Otosclerosis

◆ Hearing loss starting in early adult life; 85% bilateral; female : male ratio 2 : 1
◆ 75% also complain of tinnitus
◆ 50% have family history (autosomal dominant with incomplete penetrance)
◆ Worse in menstruation, pregnancy and menopause and improves with background noise

Cholesteatoma

◆ Invasive, non-malignant epithelial growth which often becomes infected
◆ Can be congenital or acquired, so ask about family history
◆ Progressive unilateral deafness, with repeated episodes of purulent discharge
◆ Local effects such as headache, facial nerve palsy and vertigo may also be present

Nasopharyngeal tumour

◆ Can cause Eustachian tube blockage, causing symptoms below:
  ● Gradual unilateral hearing loss. repeated infections and a feeling of fullness in the ear
  ● Local effects – headache, mandibular immobility, facial numbness and nosebleeds

Sensorineural hearing loss
Presbycusis

◆ Gradual loss of hearing starting with high-frequency sounds from age 30 years
◆ Normally occurs in both ears, but can be to different extents
◆ Worse with background noise or when multiple people are speaking
◆ Not normally a problem until later life, when certain high-frequency vocal sounds cannot be heard

Ménière's disease

◆ Progressive deafness
◆ Attacks of vertigo with nausea, tinnitus and a feeling of ear fullness occur in clusters
◆ Associated with high-salt diets and alcohol, caffeine and tobacco consumption

Other causes of hearing loss

◆ Sudden sensorineural loss can be due to numerous causes (surgical sieve) and requires prompt ENT referral and investigation
◆ Medications ('Voices More Quiet')
◆ Post-infectious ('HIS MMM')
◆ Environmental (noise)
◆ Multiple sclerosis
◆ Malignancy – acoustic neuroma, metastases or another primary brain tumour
◆ Stroke (rare)
◆ Vasculitis (rare)

Investigations

- Full neurological and ENT examination with Rinne's and Weber's tests
- Otoscopy
- Pure-tone audiometry
- Bloods – gentamicin level (if relevant), FBC, U&Es, LFTs, CRP and ESR
- Evoked-response audiometry
- CT/MRI
- Biopsy of nasopharyngeal lesions and local lymph nodes

Management

- Review medications, e.g. gentamicin and general measures, e.g. avoiding loud concerts and any occupational hazards where possible
- Ear wax – ear drops (e.g. olive oil); irrigation or microsuction if available
- Glue ear – watchful waiting; consider adenoidectomy and grommets (e.g. if prolonged history, > 3 months)
- Tympanic membrane perforation – watchful waiting; antibiotics if infected; tympanoplasty if symptomatic and fails to heal by itself
- Otosclerosis – surgery – stapedectomy or stapedotomy; hearing aids
- Cholesteatoma – surgery to remove cholesteatoma and topical antibiotics
- Ménière's disease – inform DVLA; anti-emetics for acute attacks; prophylaxis – avoid caffeine, alcohol and tobacco; prophylactic betahistine; hearing aids

Psychiatry

Low mood/depression 126

Anxiety 129

Hallucinations/delusions 133

Forgetfulness 136

Mania 140

Alcohol history 143

Eating disorder 147

Self-harm/suicide attempt (risk
assessment) 150

Low mood/depression

HPC

- Can you tell me more about this?
- How long have you felt like this? How have things progressed?
- Can you think of any reason for feeling like this? How did it all start?
- How has this affected you?

Core symptoms

- **Low mood** – How have you been feeling in yourself recently?
- **Anhedonia** – Are you able to get enjoyment from anything?
- **Fatigue** – How are your energy levels?

Other common symptoms

- **Sleep** – Are you sleeping OK? Do you wake up earlier than you used to? How much earlier?
- **Appetite** – How is your appetite? Do you think you have lost any weight?
- **Libido** – How is your libido?
- **Diurnal variation** – Does your mood change at all during the day?
- **Concentration** – Are you able to concentrate when watching TV?
- **Self** – How do you feel about yourself right now? Do you feel worthless at all? Guilty?
- **Future/hopelessness** – How do you feel about the future?

Risk – *consider a mini-summary just before this point*

- It sounds like things have become very difficult for you lately. Has it ever got so bad that you thought of harming yourself or others? *If yes, conduct full risk assessment* (*see* Self harm/suicide attempt, p. 150)

Ruling out other diagnoses

- **Hypothyroidism** – You mentioned you have put on weight (*signposting*). Do you feel cold even when others say they are warm? *If yes, ask about other symptoms* (*e.g. menstrual abnormalities, dry puffy skin, hair thinning*)
- **Bipolar** – Have you ever felt so good that other people said you were 'hyper' and not yourself?
- **Psychosis** – Have you ever seen or heard things you couldn't quite explain?
- **Anxiety** – Do you ever feel particularly worried or anxious about anything?

PMH

- Do you suffer from any medical conditions or psychiatric conditions? *If yes, how long have you suffered from this for?*
- *Ask specifically about thyroid disease, depression, mania and schizophrenia*
- How would someone close to you have described you 2 years ago?

DH

- Are you taking any prescribed medications?
- Do you have any allergies?

FH
+ Do any conditions run in your family?
+ *Ask specifically about depression and psychiatric illness generally*

SH
+ Are you currently working? If so, what is your job?
+ Who is at home? Do you have family or friends to support you?
+ Do you smoke? How many cigarettes do you smoke a day? For how long have you smoked?
+ Do you drink alcohol? How much do you drink in a week?
+ Do you take any recreational drugs?

To finish
+ **Insight and support** – From what we have discussed, I feel you are suffering from depression. Do you agree? There is support and therapy available. Is this something you would be interested in talking about?
+ **Follow-up** – I would like to see you again. Can we arrange a time to meet, perhaps next week? We could then discuss how to go forward from here

Important points
+ Be empathetic to the patient's concerns and how the symptoms have affected them. Good communication skills are particularly important in histories like this one
+ Be sure to ask about past manic episodes and alcohol consumption as well as ruling out organic causes such as hypothyroidism
+ As with all psychiatric histories, never forget to properly assess risk
+ There is less chance of further suicide attempts in the immediate future if the patient has something to look forward to, so offer an early follow-up appointment

Differential diagnosis
In a pressurised situation and with only a short time to take the history, remembering to consider differential diagnoses for low mood can be easily forgotten. It is, however, very important not to fall into the trap of simply labelling the patient with depression without due consideration of the differentials. A few simple questions can ensure you have the correct diagnosis in mind. Dual diagnoses are common in psychiatry, so also consider the possibility of coexisting schizophrenia and anxiety. As well as those listed below, sleep-related disorders, dehydration and side effects of drugs such as beta blockers can also cause low mood, whilst anaemia may primarily cause fatigue.

Depression
+ Core symptoms – low mood, anhedonia and fatigue
+ Typical symptoms – sleep disturbance, early morning waking (> 2 hours earlier than usual), decreased appetite, weight loss (> 10%), decreased libido,

diurnal mood variation, feelings of worthlessness, guilt and hopelessness, decreased concentration and attention; recurrent thoughts of death/suicide
+ Symptoms must be present for at least 2 weeks

Bipolar disorder
+ Easy-to-miss diagnosis in OSCEs – don't forget to ask about previous manic episodes
+ Symptoms of mania include euphoria, grandiosity, flight of ideas, pressure of speech and a reduced need for sleep

Schizoaffective disorder
+ Ask about delusions and hallucinations

Hypothyroidism
+ If time, ask one simple screening question, e.g. regarding intolerance of the cold
+ Other symptoms include constipation, oligomenorrhoea and weight gain

Investigations
+ Mental state examination
+ Risk assessment
+ Assess hydration status and perform thyroid exam
+ FBC and TFTs

Management
Mild
+ Regular exercise
+ Advice on sleep hygiene (regular sleep times, appropriate environment)
+ Psychosocial therapy – CBT

Moderate–severe
+ Regular exercise, advice on sleep hygiene, CBT
+ Medication – SSRIs
+ High-intensity psychosocial intervention (CBT or interpersonal therapy)
+ Immediate and considerable high risk to themselves or others:
  • Admit to psychiatric ward (use Mental Health Act if necessary)

Anxiety

PC

1. Worried or fearful, either generally or in a specific situation
2. Episode(s) of chest pain, palpitations/heart racing, nausea, etc.

HPC

NB: this will primarily concentrate on the first presenting complaint. A history for the second presenting complaint requires greater attention to organic (e.g. cardio-respiratory) causes as the primary concern (see Cardiorespiratory medicine, p. 51)

 ♦ **Open question** – Can you tell me a bit more about what has been happening?
 ♦ **Onset** – When did it all start?
 ♦ **Progression** – How has it progressed?
 ♦ **Triggers** – Did anything happen that may have started it off?
 ♦ **Description** – Can you describe to me exactly what it is like when these worries come on?
 ♦ **Symptoms** – Have you noticed getting a dry mouth when this happens? Sweating? Tremor? Sickly feeling? Awareness of your heart beating quickly? Pain anywhere? Can you describe this pain to me?
 ♦ **Severity** – I can see this is really troubling you. How is it affecting your life?

ICE

 ♦ What do you think is going on? Is there anything in particular you would like to discuss?

Diagnostic questions

 ♦ **Panic attack** – Are you ever overcome by sudden feelings of panic that seem to hit you out of the blue? What happens exactly? How long does it last?
 ♦ **Phobia** – Is there a particular time, place or situation where these feelings come on?
 ♦ **Generalised anxiety disorder** – Do you feel on edge all the time? Would you describe yourself as a worrier?
 ♦ **Obsessive–compulsive disorder** – Do you get repetitive intrusive thoughts which you cannot resist? If so, what happens when you get these thoughts? Do you have any rituals or routines that you feel compelled to follow? If so, how would you feel if you did not follow them?
 ♦ **Depression with secondary anxiety** – Do you ever feel low in mood? Do you think you could be depressed?
 ♦ **Hyperthyroidism** – Have you noticed any change in your weight or appetite? Any change in the regularity or intensity of your periods?

Risk

 ♦ I'm sorry, but it is important that I ask this. Have you ever had any thoughts of harming yourself?

PMH

- How was your childhood growing up? Do you have any traumatic memories?
- How would someone close to you have described you a few years ago? If relevant, have you always been a worrier?
- Do you suffer from any medical or psychiatric conditions?
- *Ask specifically about hypertension, angina, atrial fibrillation, hyperthyroidism and diabetes*

DH

- Are you currently taking any medication?
- How would you feel about taking medication to help if we felt it was appropriate?
- Are you allergic to any medications?

FH

- Do any conditions run in your family?
- Has anyone else in your family suffered from similar problems?

SH

- Are you currently working?
- Who is at home? Do you have family or friends to support you?
- Do you smoke? How many cigarettes do you smoke a day? For how long have you smoked?
- Do you drink alcohol? How much do you drink in a week?
- Do you use any recreational drugs?

Important points

- Must rule out organic causes – always consider if it could be cardiac in origin
- In histories such as this, your communication skills are vitally important to obtaining a good mark – build rapport with the patient and start the history empathetically, e.g. 'I can see you're upset. It must have been difficult for you to come here today.' How has this affected their life? Some patients simply cannot function at all with anxiety, and even seeing the doctor could be a horrible trauma to them
- It is difficult/impossible to do a full history for anxiety in less than 10 minutes, but if you have time, asking about their childhood may reveal events that could have drastically influenced their present state

Differential diagnosis

The most important aspect of this history is to make sure the symptoms don't have an organic cause. If in any doubt, spend more time asking them questions regarding the cardiorespiratory systems in particular. If you spend all your time asking anxiety-related questions and the patient actually has an arrhythmia, then your chances of passing this particular station will not be high.

General symptoms of an anxiety disorder

- Autonomic arousal – palpitations, sweating, tremor, dry mouth
- Chest and abdominal symptoms – breathing difficulty, feeling of choking, chest pain, nausea or abdominal distress (e.g. churning in stomach)
- Symptoms involving mental state – feeling dizzy or fearful
- General symptoms – hot flushes, cold chills, numbness, restlessness, feeling tense or irritable

Generalised anxiety disorder

- Feeling tense and worried by everyday situations
- Symptoms must have been present for at least 6 months
- The anxiety cannot be due to a physical disorder such as hyperthyroidism

Panic attack

- Unpredictable recurrent episodes of severe anxiety
- Sudden onset and lasts a few minutes
- Not associated with marked exertion or exposure to dangerous situations

Phobic anxiety disorders (agoraphobia, social and specific phobias)

- Anxiety evoked by particular situations leading to significant emotional distress
- Subsequent avoidance of these particular situations
- Includes a panic attack which occurs in an established phobic situation
- Agoraphobia includes fears of leaving home, public places, crowds, travelling alone
- Social phobia is a fear of scrutiny by others and consequently social situations
- Specific phobias are phobias restricted to highly specific situations (e.g. heights or flying)

Acute stress reaction

- Develops quickly after an unexpected life crisis
- Symptoms settle within hours–days

Post-traumatic stress disorder

- Develops weeks–months after the trauma of a threatening or catastrophic event (e.g. a life-threatening situation or sexual abuse)
- Typical features include flashbacks, nightmares, detachment, anxiety, depression and avoiding anything that may trigger memories of the trauma

Cardiogenic causes

- Angina/ACS – crushing central chest pain radiating to arm/jaw on exertion
- Atrial fibrillation – palpitations and shortness of breath (typical anxiety symptoms unlikely)

Hyperthyroidism
- Non-specific symptoms include anxiety, tremor, sweating, palpitations, irritability
- Weight loss despite increased appetite, oligomenorrhoea, diarrhoea, ophthalmopathy and a goitre all indicate a diagnosis of hyperthyroidism

Alcohol withdrawal
- Causes non-specific symptoms of anxiety, nausea, sweating, tremor and irritability
- In severe form, delirium tremens, hallucinations, fever and seizures may occur
- History of alcohol abuse is imperative to making diagnosis

Hypoglycaemia
- Most commonly seen in diabetics with mistakes in timing or amount of insulin taken

Investigations
- Physical examination to look for signs of hyperthyroidism and cardiac disease
- Bloods – TFTs and glucose
- Blood pressure (phaeochromocytoma – rare)

Management
- Counselling
- Psychotherapy – CBT
- Relaxation training
- Medication – beta blockers and SSRIs

Hallucinations/delusions

PC

1. Patient presenting with another complaint (e.g. headache) who you notice is acting strangely (they may have seemingly delusional thoughts, appear dishevelled and agitated or even respond to their hallucinations during the consultation)
2. Brought in by the police
3. Brought in by friends and/or family

HPC

+ I understand you have been under a lot of stress recently. Sometimes when people are under stress, they can have strange or unusual experiences. What I mean by that is they can hear voices, see things or feel paranoid
+ Have you had any of these experiences yourself? What have you noticed?
+ When did you first notice this? How have things progressed?

Auditory hallucinations

+ **Open question** – Can you tell me about the voices? How many are there?
+ **True/false** – Where do you hear them – inside or outside your head?
+ Can you ever stop them?
+ **Second/third person** – Do they talk to you or about you?
+ **Commands** – Do they ask you to do things? *If so*, what do they ask you to do?
+ **Running commentary** – Do you hear them like a running commentary?

Other hallucinations (visual, gustatory, olfactory)

+ **Visual** – Do you see things which others can't? *If so*, can you describe them to me? When did you first notice this? How have things progressed since?
+ **Gustatory/olfactory** – Have you noticed any strange tastes or smells that you couldn't explain? When did this start? How have things progressed?

Delusions

+ **Persecutory** – Do you feel anyone is out to get you?
+ **Reference** – Does the newspaper, radio or television refer to you?
+ **Control** – Is anyone trying to control you?
+ **Passivity** – Is anyone trying to control your actions or feelings?
+ **Grandiose** – Do you feel you have any special powers or abilities?
+ **Nihilistic** – Do you feel your organs are rotting?

Whatever the type of delusion, ask about how long it has been going on for and check the fixity by gently challenging it (e.g. 'How sure are you about that?').

Ruling out other psychiatric diagnoses

+ How has your mood been? Have you ever been diagnosed with depression, mania or anxiety?

Risk assessment

+ I can see you have clearly been under a lot of stress recently. Have things ever got so bad that you've thought of harming yourself at all? Have things ever reached a stage where you have thought of harming others?

PMH
+ Do you suffer from any medical or psychiatric conditions?

DH
+ Are you currently taking any medications?
+ Do you have any allergies?

FH
+ Do any conditions run in your family?
+ *Ask specifically about psychiatric disorders*

SH
+ Do you drink alcohol? Do you smoke? How much?
+ Are you currently employed? If so, what is your job? What effect has everything had on your job?
+ Who is at home with you? Do you have much support from friends and family?

To finish
+ **Insight** – If I were to say as a doctor I thought you had a psychiatric problem, how would you feel about that? Would you take treatment for this if a psychiatrist felt it was appropriate?

Important points
+ Offer plenty of reassurance and empathy before firing questions
+ Try to connect with your patient's symptoms
+ If presenting with a headache or other complaint, be sure to ask relevant questions about that complaint first, as even psychiatric patients can get ill!

Differential diagnosis
Schizophrenia
+ Schneider's first-rank symptoms – auditory hallucinations, delusions of perception, delusions of control and thought echo, insertion, withdrawal and broadcasting
+ Negative symptoms – anhedonia, blunting of responses, poverty of speech and marked apathy
+ Positive symptoms – hallucinations of any modality, catatonia, neologisms and tangential speech
+ Risk factors include family history, heavy cannabis use and social isolation
+ High risk of suicide, so always assess risk

Drug-induced psychosis
◆ Many drugs, including alcohol, cannabis and LSD, can either mimic psychosis through intoxication or cause a chronic hallucinosis in long-term misuse
◆ Withdrawal states such as delirium tremens can also mimic psychosis

Delirium
◆ An acute confusional state common in the elderly
◆ Can be the mode of presentation for infection in the elderly (e.g. UTI)
◆ Other causes include drugs (e.g. morphine, steroids and benzodiazepines), alcohol abuse/withdrawal, metabolic disturbances and stroke

Depression with psychosis
◆ Core features of depression present (low mood, anhedonia and fatigue)
◆ Delusions are the most common psychotic symptoms in depression (e.g. delusions of guilt, paranoia, persecution and nihilism)
◆ Patient may believe they are being punished for previous wrongs or that they are responsible for acts which they clearly could not be responsible for
◆ Hallucinations may involve hearing voices that are heavily critical of them

Mania
◆ Signs and symptoms include elated mood, high energy levels and self-esteem, grandiosity, flight of ideas and restlessness
◆ Delusions of grandiosity are often present, as may other delusions (e.g. persecutory) or even hallucinations
◆ Patient will be talking very fast, constantly switching between topics
◆ There may be a previous history of depression (bipolar disorder)

Investigations
◆ Full physical examination, including neurological examination
◆ Mental state examination
◆ Bloods – FBC, U&Es , LFTs, TFTs, vitamin B_{12}, blood glucose and folate
◆ Urine drug screen
◆ Chest X-ray
◆ If indicated – serology for syphilis, lumbar puncture, EEG and MRI/CT brain

Management
◆ Biopsychosocial approach
◆ Psychological treatment – psychotherapy and CBT
◆ Psychosocial rehabilitation – psychoeducation; social worker (finances)
◆ Pharmacological treatment – oral or intramuscular second-generation (atypical) antipsychotic (e.g. risperidone or olanzapine)
◆ Treatment can be given in both outpatient or inpatient setting
◆ Inpatient setting indicated when patient is high risk to self or others – use of the Mental Health Act may be necessary
◆ Community follow-up and close working with patient and family
◆ Electroconvulsive therapy can be used in catatonic schizophrenia

Forgetfulness

HPC

◆ When did you first notice this? How did you notice it?
◆ How has it progressed?

Cognition

◆ **Short-term memory** – Do you have any difficulty remembering names? Appointments? Dates? Do you remember to take your medications every day?
◆ **Long-term memory** – Can you remember when you got married? What was your first job?
◆ **Visuospatial difficulties** – Do you have any difficulty recognising places, people or any items?
◆ **Language** – Do you ever struggle to find the right words when talking?

Changes

◆ **Behaviour** – Have you noticed any change in your behaviour? (*E.g. irritability, sexual disinhibition, wandering and social withdrawal*)
◆ **Personality** – Have you noticed any changes in your personality? (*E.g. violence/outbursts, verbal/physical aggression*)

Ruling out other psychiatric diagnoses

◆ **Depression** – How is your mood?
◆ **Anxiety** – Have you been feeling upset or anxious recently?
◆ **Psychosis** – I know this may sound silly, but have you seen or heard things that you couldn't quite explain?

Ruling out organic causes

◆ **Constitutional** – Have you been feeling ill or poorly recently? Any fever?
◆ **Parkinsonism** – Have you noticed a tremor in either hand at all? Have you noticed any changes in your walking? Any changes in your handwriting?

Risk assessment

◆ **Coping with activities of daily living** – Tell me about your current home situation. Are you coping? Are you able to wash yourself regularly? Dress yourself? Do the cleaning? Cooking? Shopping? How are things financially?
◆ **Dangerous events** – Have you had any falls? Have your neighbours or friends ever found you wandering the streets looking confused?
◆ **Driving** – Do you drive? If so, have you ever had any near-accidents? If so, what happened?
◆ **Harm** – I know things have been difficult recently, but have they ever got so bad that you've thought about harming yourself or others?

PMH

◆ Do you suffer from any medical or psychiatric conditions?
◆ *Ask specifically about problems hearing and visual difficulties*

DH

♦ Are you currently taking any medications? Do you remember to take them every day?
♦ Do you have any allergies?

FH

♦ Do any conditions run in your family?
♦ *Ask specifically about dementia*

SH

♦ Do you smoke? Do you drink alcohol? How much?
♦ Do you currently work or have you retired? *If working,* how has this affected your job?
♦ Do you have a husband/wife? Children? Grandchildren? Are your family able to offer much support?

To finish

♦ **Collateral history** – Thank you for talking to me. I would like to talk to one of your close family or friends who has been concerned about you to ask them some questions. Is that OK with you?

Important points

♦ It is very important to rule out organic causes of dementia, as these may be reversible
♦ You must assess the ability of the patient to cope in day-to-day living and fully assess risk
♦ Does the patient have any support from family, friends or neighbours? If not, consider whether they might need further care offered

Differential diagnosis

Alzheimer's disease

♦ Progressive global impairment of cognitive functioning
♦ Short-term memory often affected first, followed by confusion, irritability, aggression, long-term memory loss, mood swings and incontinence
♦ Most common form of dementia, accounting for over half of cases
♦ Risk factors include advanced age, Caucasian race, female sex and vascular disease

Vascular dementia

♦ Stepwise decline in cognitive functioning over months–years
♦ Evidence of previous stroke with onset of dementia within 3 months of stroke
♦ Cardiovascular risk factor likely to be present

Dementia with Lewy bodies

♦ Fluctuating confusion
♦ Parkinsonian features (e.g. tremor, bradykinesia, festinating gait and ataxia

leading to falls and micrographia), visual hallucinations and intermittent loss of consciousness
◆ Short-term memory often preserved to a greater extent than in Alzheimer's, but visuospatial difficulties are more pronounced

Frontotemporal dementia
◆ Aggression, inappropriate social behaviour, emotional blunting, incontinence and speech and language difficulties all tend to occur early
◆ Often insidious, with an earlier age of onset than in Alzheimer's disease

Other causes (including organic)
◆ Normal ageing process – impairment of memory and intellect is common in the elderly, but does not always justify a diagnosis of dementia!
◆ Delirium – acute confusional state common in the elderly, often due to infection, drugs (e.g. morphine) or alcohol
◆ Depressive pseudodementia – common in elderly; often present with memory impairment and difficulty in attention and concentration
◆ Metabolic disturbances – e.g. uraemia from renal or liver failure, hypothyroidism, hypo-/hypercalcaemia, hypoglycaemia and vitamin B_{12} deficiency
◆ Brain tumour – behavioural/personality changes, headaches, seizures and nausea and vomiting are common features; usually a secondary tumour
◆ Parkinson's disease – Parkinsonian features preceding symptoms of dementia by at least 1 year

Investigations
Note: It is of paramount importance in dementia to rule out organic causes.
◆ Full physical examination, including thyroid status
◆ Mini mental state examination
◆ Bloods – FBC, U&Es, LFTs, TFTs, vitamin B_{12}, blood glucose and folate
◆ Blood cultures
◆ Chest X-ray
◆ EEG
◆ MRI/CT brain
◆ Lumbar puncture (if Creutzfeldt–Jakob disease suspected)
◆ If needed – serology for syphilis, PET scan and DAT scan

Management
◆ Treat the underlying cause (if treatable) – e.g. management of thyroid disease, B_{12} deficiency, shunting in hydrocephalus, levodopa in Parkinson's, etc.
◆ Symptomatic – environmental manipulation; lifestyle factors, e.g. exercise, reduce alcohol and smoking, and encourage reading
◆ Supportive care for the family (including social worker input) – caring for people with dementia is very demanding and can place a lot of stress on families; it is important to ensure the carer is being followed up him/herself
◆ Alzheimer's disease – memory-enhancing drugs, e.g. rivastigmine

- ◆ Advice from DVLA after diagnosis of dementia
- ◆ Late stages of dementia – residential or nursing homes may be the last option

Mania
PC
1. 'I feel on top of the world, doctor!'
2. 'My partner has been upset for some reason and dragged me here, but I feel great, doctor, and have so many things to do . . .'

HPC
+ **Clarify** – Can I just check what you mean by that/what your partner was worried about?
+ **Open question** – Tell me, how have things been recently?
+ **Reflect** – *Reflect on the manic features as you notice them – spell it out for your half-asleep examiner!*
+ **Onset** – How long have you felt like this?

Key features
+ **Elated mood** – How are you feeling in yourself? How is your mood on a scale of 1–10? *Patient most likely will have already volunteered this information!*
+ **High energy levels** – How are your energy levels?
+ **High self-esteem** – How would you describe your self-esteem?
+ **Grandiosity** – Do you have any special powers or abilities? Can you communicate with God? Do you think you can fly? *If yes, risk-assess*
+ **Flight of ideas** (*reflect back to the patient if he is very talkative and switching topics mid-conversation without letting you get a word in!*)

Biological
+ **Restlessness** – How is your sleep? ('*I don't have time to sleep*')
+ **Poor appetite** – How is your appetite? ('*I eat when I feel hungry, but I don't have time to eat*')
+ **Increased libido** – How is your sex drive? Do you have a regular partner? Have you slept with anyone else recently? Have you ever paid for sex?

Risk assessment
+ **Overspending** – Do you ever go on shopping binges? How are things financially?
+ **Police** – Have you got into any trouble with the police recently? If so, why?
+ **Self-harm/suicide** – Have you ever tried to harm yourself? Have you ever tried to use your special power(s)? If so, what happened?

Ruling out other diagnoses
+ **Bipolar** – I know you feel great now, but have you ever been depressed?
+ **Anxiety** – Do you ever feel particularly worried or anxious about anything?
+ **Psychosis** – Have you ever seen or heard things that you couldn't quite explain?

PMH

+ Have you ever been diagnosed with any medical or psychiatric conditions?
+ *Ask specifically about thyroid disease, depression and psychosis*

DH

+ Do you take any medications?
+ Do you have any allergies?

FH

+ Do any conditions run in your family?

SH

+ Do you drink alcohol? How much do you drink in a week? Do you binge-drink?
+ Do you use any recreational drugs? When did you start? What do you use?
+ Do you smoke? How many do you smoke in a week? For how many years?
+ Are you currently employed? If not, why and what was your last job?
+ Have your family and friends been upset by any of your behaviour recently? If so, can you tell me why? How does your partner feel about what's been happening?

Important points

+ A manic patient might be very talkative during the interview. It is best not to interrupt them in the first 1–2 minutes, but it may be necessary after this due to time constraints, e.g. 'I'm sorry to interrupt you, but can I please ask ...'
+ Alternatively, in a difficult scenario, the patient may have some control over his or her symptoms and try to appear normal after being forced to come by his or her family/friends – here, taking a collateral history is particularly important
+ The best way to show to the examiner that you can elicit the mania history is to reflect back to the patient:
  + If the patient is talking rapidly – 'You seem to talk quite fast' (pressured speech)
  + If the patient is saying lots of things, jumping from topic to topic – 'You seem to have lots of ideas' (flight of ideas)
  + If the patient says they can talk to God – 'You seem to have special powers'

Differential diagnosis

Mania

+ Signs and symptoms include elated mood, high energy levels and self-esteem, grandiosity, flight of ideas and restlessness
+ Patient will be talking very fast, constantly switching between topics
+ Patient engages in pleasurable activities without considering negative consequences (e.g. sexual disinhibition, whilst not considering contraception)
+ Shopping sprees are often described with money the patient does not have, therefore creating large amounts of debt and sometimes involving the police

- Delusions of grandiosity are often present, as may other delusions (e.g. persecutory) or even hallucinations
- Can have profound effect upon relationships with friends and family

Hypomania
- Persistent, milder form of mania, with slightly elevated mood that alternates with irritability, high energy levels and restlessness
- Delusions and hallucinations are not present

Bipolar affective disorder
- Manic symptoms in a patient with a previous history of depression

Schizoaffective disorder
- Significant history of manic and/or depressive episodes concurrent with symptoms of schizophrenia
- Schneider's first-rank symptoms – auditory hallucinations, delusions of perception, delusions of control and thought echo, insertion, withdrawal and broadcasting
- Risk factors include family history, heavy cannabis use and social isolation

Drug-induced psychosis
- Many drugs, including alcohol, cannabis and LSD, can either mimic psychosis through intoxication or cause a chronic hallucinosis in long-term misuse
- Withdrawal states such as delirium tremens can also mimic psychosis

Adjustment disorder
- Insomnia, poor concentration, avoiding important jobs, skipping school/work are signs that may mimic mania
- Low mood and anxiety in the context of an identifiable stressor help distinguish the disorder from other diagnoses

Investigations
- Physical examination, including assessment for a goitre
- Mental state examination
- Bloods – FBC, U&Es , LFTs, TFTs, vitamin B_{12}, blood glucose and folate
- Urine drug screen
- Chest X-ray
- If indicated – lumbar puncture and MRI/CT brain

Management
- Biopsychosocial approach
- Psychological – CBT, interpersonal therapy and family therapy
- Psychoeducation and vocational rehabilitation
- Pharmacological – mood stabilizers, e.g. lithium; antipsychotics (e.g. olanzapine); benzodiazepines (e.g. lorazepam) to help insomnia/restlessness;

antidepressants only used in selected cases, as they can induce a manic episode
- Treatment can be given in both outpatient or inpatient setting
- Inpatient setting indicated when patient is high risk to self or others

Alcohol history
PC
1. 'My wife thinks I have a problem with alcohol and made me see you today . . .'
2. 'I was struck off work recently, and things have been deteriorating since . . .'
3. 'I think I'm developing a problem with alcohol . . .'

HPC
Drinking pattern
+ Can you tell me about your drinking?
+ Starting from first thing in the morning, talk me through what you drink in a typical day
+ **What** do you drink?
+ **How much** do you drink?
+ **When** do you start?
+ **Where** do you drink?
+ **Alone** – Do you drink alone?
+ **Progression** – How has your drinking progressed?

CAGE questionnaire
+ **Cut down** – Have you ever felt you should Cut down on your drinking?
+ **Annoy** – Do people Annoy you by criticising your drinking?
+ **Guilty** – Do you feel Guilty about your drinking?
+ **Eye-opener** – Do you drink first think in the morning?

Features of dependence
+ **Tolerance** – Do you have to drink more to get the same effect you used to?
+ **Withdrawal** –What happens when you don't drink? Do you get shakes or sweats when you don't drink for a few days?
+ **Compulsion** – Do you get any cravings or urges for alcohol?
+ **Primacy** – Would you say drinking has become your main priority in life?
+ **Previous treatment** – Have you ever had any treatments or detox for alcohol? What helped? What triggered your relapse?

Consequences
+ Has your drinking caused any problems in your life?
+ How has your drinking affected your **working life**? How are things financially for you at the moment?
+ How has your drinking affected your **relationships** with friends and family?
+ Have you had any problems with the **law**? Do you ever drive after drinking?

Complications
+ **Physical complications** – Have you noticed any weight loss? How is your appetite? Have you had any problems with your memory?
+ **Depression/anxiety** – How has your mood been over the past few weeks?
+ **Psychosis** – Have you noticed any strange or unusual experiences?

- **Self-harm/suicide** – It seems as if things have been very difficult for you recently. Have things ever got so bad that you thought about harming yourself?

PMH
- Do you suffer from any medical or psychiatric conditions?
- Ask specifically about diabetes, liver disease and cardiovascular disease

DH
- Are you currently taking any medications?
- Do you have any allergies?

FH
- Has anyone in your family had problems with alcohol?
- Do any conditions run in your family?

SH
- Do you smoke?
- Do you use any recreational drugs?

Insight
It seems alcohol has been a significant part of your life . . .
- Do you think you have a drink problem?
- Do you want to stop or reduce your drinking?
- Would you be interested in accepting help if offered to you?

Important points
- It is important to develop a rapport with the patient before asking personal questions about their drinking habits – otherwise patients are likely to be resistive and potentially dishonest in answering your questioning
- The CAGE questionnaire, whilst a useful screening tool, should not be used as a substitute for a full alcohol history
- It is important to take a holistic approach to an alcohol history – it is important to know what affect alcohol has had on their life, just as it is important to find any potential complications arising from alcohol abuse
- Never forget to assess risk in a psychiatric history
- A similar approach can be used when taking a recreational drug history

Differential diagnosis
Alcoholism is suggested by all the features listed in bold in this history. Differentials for this history are not relevant, as the key aspect is to see whether the candidate can ascertain all the important information about the patient's drinking.

Investigations

- General physical examination, involving assessing for malnourishment, signs of liver disease and signs of heart disease (including atrial fibrillation and alcoholic cardiomyopathy)
- Bloods – FBC (macrocytic anaemia), U&Es, CRP, LFTs, clotting screen, lipids, glucose, gamma-GT and vitamin levels (particularly thiamine)
- In acute state of intoxication, also measure blood alcohol levels
- Further investigations depend on any related illness, e.g. abdominal ultrasound and CT/MRI abdomen (for liver disease) and echocardiography (for heart disease)

Management

General measures

- Advice about the adverse effects of alcohol
- Vitamin supplements, including thiamine to prevent Wernicke's encephalopathy
- Support and advice (including a listening ear at times)
- Financial support where possible and indicated

Acute alcohol withdrawal

- Consider whether the patient needs inpatient management
- IV Pabrinex or oral thiamine to prevent Wernicke's encephalopathy
- Chlordiazepoxide to treat tremor and agitation in delirium tremens

Abstinence

- Social support – involve family and friends in their care where possible
- Support groups, including Alcoholics Anonymous or similar groups
- CBT
- Acamprosate – reduces cravings
- Naltrexone – reduces pleasurable effects of alcohol; particularly effective in binge drinkers
- Disulfiram – causes an unpleasant reaction if the patient drinks alcohol, including nausea, headache and palpitations

Eating disorder

PC

1. 'I don't know why I've been dragged here, everything is fine . . .'
   - Can I ask who brought you here today?
   - What are they worried about?
2. 'Mum brought me in because she thinks I'm not eating . . .'
   - Why do you think she is worried about you?
3. 'I was wondering if there was anything you could do to help me lose some weight?'
   - Can I ask why it is you wish to lose weight?

HPC

- **Open questions** – What makes your mum/dad/friend, etc. worry about your eating? Can you tell me a bit more about your eating?
- **Typical day** – Can you describe what you eat in a typical day, starting from the morning?
- **Bingeing** – Do you ever binge on food? If yes, how do you feel afterwards? Do you do anything to counteract the binge? What do you do? Do you ever deliberately make yourself sick afterwards or use laxatives?
- **Onset** – How long has this been going on for?
- **Trigger** – Did anything bring it on?
- **Home environment** – How are things at home?

SCOFF questions – *recognised screening tool for eating disorders*

Would you mind, for your mum's sake, if I asked some quick questions about your eating?

- **Sick** – Do you make yourself *Sick* because you are uncomfortably full?
- **Control** – Do you worry that you have lost *Control* over how much you eat?
- **One stone** – Have you lost more than 6 kg (about *One stone*) in the past 3 months?
- **Feel fat** – Do you believe you are *Fat* even when others think you are thin?
- **Food dominates** – Would you say that *Food* dominates your life?

WAIF questions

- **Weight** – I'm sorry, I know this is personal, but can I ask how much you weigh? How tall are you? (*NB: Is there a BMI scale/calculator in the room?*)
- **Amenorrhoea** – Have your periods been coming regularly?
- **Induced vomiting** – Have you ever made yourself throw up after eating? Do you exercise much? (How often?)
- **Fear of fatness** – How would you feel if you gained weight?

Systems review

- How are your waterworks? Bowels? Do you have any pain anywhere? Bleeding anywhere?

PMH

♦ Do you suffer from any medical or psychiatric illnesses?
♦ *Ask specifically about diabetes and hyperthyroidism*

DH

♦ Are you currently taking any medication?
♦ Are you taking anything to help lose weight, such as laxatives, water tablets or appetite suppressants? *If so*, are you aware of the dangers these can pose?
♦ Do you have any allergies?

FH

♦ Do any conditions run in the family?
♦ *Ask specifically about eating disorders and psychiatric disorders generally*

SH

♦ Do you smoke? Drink alcohol? How much?
♦ What do your friends think about your weight? Do they say anything? Are you in a relationship? What does he/she think?
♦ Are you currently working? What is your job? What effect has this had on your job?

Important points

♦ Do not jump straight in and ask them how much they weigh. This can be a very sensitive issue, and these patients are often resistive. Try to establish trust and rapport in the beginning
♦ Be sensitive and non-judgemental about how they look
♦ In the back of your mind, always consider whether there could be an organic disease

Differential diagnosis

It is very important to rule out possible organic causes if a patient is underweight. The key in eating disorders is that the patient has a distorted body image and wishes to lose weight. If they are concerned about their weight loss or their weight loss is unintended, then careful questioning into possible organic causes is needed.

Anorexia nervosa

♦ Underweight (BMI < 17.5)
♦ Distorted body image – think they are fat despite being told they are thin
♦ Food dominates thinking – very careful over what they eat; may lie when asked about food consumption
♦ May utilise other methods of weight loss such as excessive exercise (e.g. 2 hours every day), taking laxatives, diuretics or appetite suppressants
♦ Fear of gaining weight
♦ Although more commonly a feature of bulimia, vomiting can also occur in anorexia
♦ Amenorrhoea/oligomenorrhoea as hormones are affected by diet

Bulimia nervosa
- Unlike in anorexia, likely to be of normal weight or overweight
- Binge eating – repetitive episodes of eating large amounts of food
- Purging – try to counteract the fattening effect of the binge by inducing vomiting (common), taking laxatives, diuretics, extreme dieting or exercise
- Eating patterns are typically irregular
- Amenorrhoea/oligomenorrhoea may again occur
- Erosion of the teeth, continuous sore throat and reflux due to purging

Investigations
- Further detailed history and mental state examination – psychiatric comorbidities are common
- Bloods – FBC, U&Es, glucose and LFTs

Management
- Advice on healthy eating – nutrition, regular balanced meals, etc.
- Psychotherapy – CBT or interpersonal therapy
- Medication – SSRIs can help reduce urge to binge and purge; or if comorbid depression

Self-harm/suicide attempt (risk assessment)
HPC
To start
+ How are you feeling today? I understand you took some tablets last night. I'm really sorry things got that bad for you that you felt there was no other way out

Before
+ **Prior events/mood** – If you don't mind me asking, what happened before that made you feel like you had to end it all/harm yourself? Have you been feeling low for a while?
+ **Plan** – Did you plan to harm yourself? What plans did you make? How long had you been planning this for?
+ **Not to be caught** – Did you try to make sure you wouldn't get caught, like locking the door or making sure you were alone?
+ **Preparation** – Did you write a note or make a will in preparation?
+ **Told anyone?** – Did you tell anybody about it before or seek help afterwards?

During
+ **Sequence of events** – Can you talk me through exactly what happened? (*How? Where? When?*)
+ **Expectations** – Did you expect to die?
+ **Alcohol/drugs** – Were you under the influence of alcohol or drugs at the time?

After
+ **Discovery** – How were you discovered? Did you tell anyone?
+ **Anger/regret** – How do you feel about what has happened?
+ **Lingering thoughts** – Do you still have any thoughts of doing something like this again?

PMH
+ Do you suffer from any medical or psychiatric illnesses such as depression?
+ Have you ever tried to take your life or harm yourself before this?

DH
+ Are you currently taking any medication?
+ Do you have stores of any medications at home?

FH
+ Has anyone in your family ever tried to harm themselves?

SH
+ Are you currently working? What is your job? How are things at work?
+ Who is at home? Do you have a partner or kids? Do you have friends around you?

+ Do you drink alcohol? How much do you drink in a week?
+ Do you take any recreational drugs?
+ Do you think you need any help? Would you be prepared to accept any help?

To finish
+ **Follow-up** – I would like to see you again next week. Can we arrange a time to meet? Is there anything you would like to talk about?

Important points
+ Empathise and establish rapport with patient before diving into what happened
+ In the back of your mind, consider if this patient is at risk of future attempts
+ If intended suicide, did they plan and prepare the act to meet their intended outcome?
+ Did they genuinely believe it would kill them or could it be a cry for attention? Pay careful attention to the method (e.g. did they only take four paracetamol tablets?)
+ There is less risk of the patient attempting self-harm in the immediate future if they have something to look forward to

Differential diagnosis
Self-harm
+ Deliberate act of self-harm with a non-fatal outcome done in the knowledge that it is potentially harmful
+ Methods:
  - Overdose (NSAIDs most commonly; antidepressants)
  - Self-inflicted injuries (e.g. cutting self)
+ Reasons for self-harm, the 8 Cs:
  - Coping mechanism
  - Control
  - Calming/comforting
  - Cleansing (e.g. from sexual abuse)
  - Confirmation of existence
  - Creating comfortable numbness
  - Chastisement (e.g. if depressed)
  - Communication
+ Risk factors:
  - Age 16–24 years
  - Female
  - Recent stressful event
  - Personality disorder
  - Areas of high unemployment rate
+ 10% lifetime suicide risk – risk highest in weeks following act

Suicide

- Deliberate act of self-harm with a fatal outcome done in the knowledge that the act is potentially fatal
- Methods:
  - Hanging
  - Self-poisoning (are they in a profession with access to dangerous chemicals?)
  - Drug/alcohol overdose
  - Gunshot (more common in US)
- Risk factors:
  - Risk increases with age
  - Male
  - Lost job
  - Separated/divorced/widowed
  - Depression/mood disorder
  - Alcohol/drug abuse
  - Serious physical illness
- Factors increasing likeliness of future suicide attempt:
  - Immediate intent after recent escalation
  - Well-constructed plan involving a violent method or with access to means
  - Likelihood of further bad news

Investigations

- Mental state examination
- Collaborative history from family/friend

Management

- Allow them to vent their emotions
- Identify possible coping mechanisms
- Bolster self-esteem
- Explore effects their suicide would have on family and friends
- Make plans for future
- Does this patient require inpatient admission?
- Ensure adequate support at home
- Give telephone number for mental health support, with instructions if things get worse
- Remove access to means
- Regular planned follow-up

Obstetrics & gynaecology

Gynaecological history template 154
Vaginal bleeding 156
Antepartum haemorrhage 160
Vaginal discharge. 163
Subfertility 166
Urinary incontinence 169
Amenorrhoea/oligomenorrhoea 172

Gynaecological history template
PCs
- Vaginal bleeding
- Vaginal discharge
- Menstrual irregularities (menorrhagia/amenorrhoea/dysmenorrhoea)
- Pain (dysmenorrhoea/dyspareunia/lower abdominal pain)
- Subfertility
- Incontinence

For the general gynaecological history, the following components must be considered.

Menstrual history (menstRUAL)
- Is there any chance you could be pregnant? How have your periods been?
- **Regularity** – How often are your periods in terms of days? How long do they usually last for?
- **Underwear** – Do you suffer from heavy or painful periods?
- **Age at menarche** – What age were you when you had your first period?
- **Last menstrual period** – When was the first day of your last period?
- *If menopausal, establish whether they are taking hormone replacement therapy*

Vaginal bleeding (SOCRAT)
- **Site** – When and where exactly did you notice the bleeding? Is it definitely coming from the vagina?
- **Onset** – When did you first notice it?
- **Character** – How much have you noticed? Have you passed clots? What colour is it?
- **Radiation** – Do you use tampons or padding? Does it soak them?
- **Associated symptoms** – *pain, discharge, menstrual irregularities and constitutional symptoms*
- **Timing** – When do you notice the bleeding? Is it there all the time? How often have you noticed it? Could it be your period? Does it occur mid-cycle? Does it come on after sex?

Pain
- **Abdo pain** – Do you have any pain in your tummy or further down? *If so,* SOCRATES
- **Dyspareunia** – Have you had any pain during sex? *If so*, where exactly? Is it a deep pain or a pain on entering?

Discharge
- Have you noticed any discharge? Can you tell me about the discharge?
- **Onset** – When did you first notice it?
- **Colour** – What colour is the discharge?
- **Odour** – Does it have a bad smell?
- **Amount** – How much have you noticed?

Sexual history

* **Last cervical smear** – When was your last smear done?
* **Sexually active?** – Are you sexually active?
* **Partner(s)** – Is it with a regular partner or different partners?
* **Contraception/HRT** – Are you currently taking contraception/hormone replacement therapy? *Specify and check compliance*
* *Take a history of sexual encounters if relevant (e.g. discharge present)*

Obstetric history

* How many pregnancies have you had?
* Did you have any complications with any of them? Did they all carry to term?
* Were they normal deliveries?

Vaginal bleeding
HPC
O'SOCRAT
- **Open question** – Can you tell me more about the bleeding?
- **Site** – When and where exactly did you notice the bleeding? Is it definitely coming from the vagina?
- **Onset** – When did you first notice it?
- **Character** – How much have you noticed? Have you passed clots? What colour is it?
- **Radiation** – Do you use tampons or padding? Does it soak them?
- **Associated symptoms** – *see later*
- **Timing** – When do you notice the bleeding? Is it there all the time? How often have you noticed it? Could it be your period? Does it occur mid-cycle? Does it come on after sex?

ICE
- Do you have any idea what might be causing this? Is there anything you are particularly worried about or would like to discuss?

MenstRUAL history
- Is there any chance you could be pregnant? How have your periods been?
- **Regularity** – How often are your periods? How long do they usually last for?
- **Underwear** – Do you suffer from heavy or painful periods?
- **Age at menarche** – What age were you when you had your first period?
- **Last menstrual period** – When was the first day of your last period?

Lower abdominal/pelvic pain
- **Abdo pain** – Have you been experiencing any pain anywhere below your belly button? *If so, SOCRATES*
- **Dyspareunia** – Do you experience any pain during sex? *If so*, where exactly? Is it a deep pain or a pain on entering?

Sexual history
- **Last cervical smear** – When was your last smear done?
- **Sexually active?** – Are you sexually active?
- **Partner(s)** – Is it with a regular partner or different partners?
- **Contraception/HRT** – Are you currently taking contraception/hormone replacement therapy? *Specify and check compliance*

Discharge
- Other than blood, have you noticed any discharge? Can you tell me about the discharge?
- **Onset** – When did you first notice it?
- **Colour** – What colour is the discharge?
- **Odour** – Does it have a bad smell?

+ **Amount** – How much have you noticed?

ROS
+ Have you noticed any weight loss? How is your appetite? Have you been particularly tired recently? Have you been breathless at all?
+ Have you had any problems with your waterworks?

Obstetric history
+ **Gravida** – How many pregnancies have you had?
+ **Complications** – Did you have any significant problems with any of them? Did they all carry to term?

PMH
+ Have you ever suffered from any medical conditions?
+ *Ask specifically about previous cancer (particularly breast, ovarian, endometrial and cervical), STIs and bleeding disorders*

DH
+ Are you currently taking any medication?
+ Do you have any allergies?

FH
+ Do any conditions run in the family?
+ *Ask specifically about breast and ovarian cancer, and determine the age they were when they were diagnosed*

SH
+ Are you currently working?
+ Do you smoke? Drink alcohol? How much?
+ Who is at home with you?

Important points
+ This is often an embarrassing complaint for patients, so use tact and try ways to make the patient feel more comfortable talking to you – e.g. 'Often people feel embarrassed talking about this, but it is a common issue. As a health professional, I am here to help and I promise I will keep everything we talk about strictly confidential.'
+ It is extremely important to ask when their last cervical smear was performed, as well as considering constitutional symptoms, to show you are thinking about cervical and endometrial cancer as possible diagnoses – failure to do so is likely to result in a poor mark
+ Enquiring about contraceptive method(s) used and compliance is important to help establish the correct diagnosis – condoms regularly used decrease the likelihood of it being cervical cancer; hormonal contraception might suggest breakthrough bleeding, whilst intrauterine contraceptive devices introduce the possibility of an ectopic pregnancy

+ You must also establish whether there is a chance the patient could be pregnant, as this might point to a very different diagnosis (e.g. ectopic pregnancy and miscarriage)

Differential diagnosis

Differential diagnosis of a PV bleed depends on the timing of the bleed – intermenstrual, post-coital or post-menopausal. Could it even simply be their period? Do they have a bleeding disorder, or are they on anticoagulant/anti-platelet medication?

Post-coital
Cervical carcinoma

+ Infection with human papillomavirus (HPV) 16 and 18
+ History of multiple partners, STIs, smoking, missed smears, weight loss and loss of appetite
+ Can also present as intermenstrual bleeding

Cervical ectropion

+ Squamocolumnar junction extends under hormonal influence (e.g. puberty, COCP and pregnancy)
+ Red ring around cervical os on examination with speculum

Cervical polyp

+ May bleed on contact
+ Can also present as intermenstrual bleeding

Post-menopausal (PV bleeding > 12 months after last period)
Endometrial carcinoma

+ Risk factors – unopposed oestrogen exposure, obesity, old age, nulliparity, late menopause and polycystic ovarian syndrome
+ Accounts for ~10% of post-menopausal bleeding, but requires urgent investigation
+ Less commonly can present as post-coital or intermenstrual bleeding

Atrophic vaginitis

+ Dry, itchy vagina with subsequent dyspareunia
+ Urinary incontinence and recurrent UTIs
+ Very common in post-menopausal women due to low levels of oestrogen

Endometrial hyperplasia

+ Exposure to high levels of oestrogen with insufficient levels of progesterone
+ Diagnosed on endometrial biopsy or curettage
+ Significant risk factor for development of endometrial carcinoma

Intermenstrual

Some women experience light bleeding or spotting that is normal during ovulation (~day 14 of cycle). Always consider if the patient could be pregnant. Spotting may occur with implantation of the blastocyst in the uterus, but also with conditions associated with pregnancy. Breakthrough bleeding is also common in the first few months of starting a hormonal contraception.

Ectopic pregnancy

- Severe, sharp, colicky abdominal pain in a sexually active woman
- Diarrhoea and vomiting may also be present
- Rupture leads to severe pain, peritonism and shock
- Occurs ~5–12 weeks after last period
- Occurs due to fertilised ovum implanting outside uterine cavity
- Increased risk of ectopic pregnancy if using intrauterine contraceptive device

Spontaneous abortion

- Loss of pregnancy at any stage up to 24th week
- Lower abdominal cramps, passing blood clots with 'tissue'

Sexually transmitted infection

- Sexually active woman with discharge that may be smelly
- Risk factors – young/adolescent, multiple partners/new partner, unprotected sex

Investigations

- Abdominal and pelvic examination – feel for any pelvic masses
- PV examination – confirm it is a PV bleed; look for pathology
- Bloods – FBC and clotting
- Urine beta-hCG (pregnancy test)
- STI screen – high vaginal and endocervical swabs
- Cervical smear (if due/overdue for smear)
- Colposcopy after abnormal smear
- Transvaginal USS
- Urgent USS if suspect ectopic pregnancy

Management

- Urgent referral for PMB or IMB/PCB if suspicion arises from PV exam
- Atrophic vaginitis – topical lubricant/cream or HRT (topical or systemic)
- Polyps – remove and send for histology
- Ectopic pregnancy – surgical intervention (either laparoscopic or open)
- STI – appropriate antibiotic treatment

Antepartum haemorrhage

HPC

O'SOCRAT

+ **Open question** – Can you tell me about what's been going on? How far along is the pregnancy?
+ **Site** – When and where exactly do you notice the bleeding? Is it definitely coming from the vagina?
+ **Onset** – When did you first notice the bleeding?
+ **Character** – How much have you noticed? What colour is it? Have you passed clots or anything odd?
+ **Radiation** – Have you had to use padding? Does it soak them?
+ **Associated symptoms** – Have you had any diarrhoea or vomiting? Any pain?
+ **Timing** – Is the bleeding there all the time? How often have you noticed it?

Present pregnancy

+ **Foetal well-being** – Have you felt the baby moving recently? Have you had any pain down below or in your tummy? *If so*, SOCRATES
+ **Last menstrual period** – When was the first day of your last period?
+ **Regularity** – Were your periods always regular? (*Could this be a period?*)
+ **Progress** – How has the pregnancy gone previous to this? Have you been suffering from high blood pressure, water infections or anything else?
+ **Tests** – What tests have been performed so far?

Past obstetric history

+ **Gravida** – Is this your first pregnancy? *Take history of each pregnancy in chronological order*
+ **Complications** – Have you had any complications during any of the pregnancies? Have you suffered any miscarriages, stillbirths or terminations?
+ **Gestational age** – How many weeks' gestation was your baby at delivery?
+ **Delivery** – How was he delivered? *If by Caesarean section*, why was this needed?
+ **Birthweight** – What was his birthweight?

ICE

+ Can I ask what you think might be going on? Obviously, this must be a worrying situation for you, but is there anything in particular you would like to discuss?

PMH

+ Do you suffer from any medical conditions?
+ *Ask specifically about bleeding disorders, lupus (antiphospholipid syndrome predisposes to recurrent miscarriages), hypertension and diabetes*

DH
♦ Are you taking any medications? (*Are any of them contraindicated in pregnancy?*)
♦ Do you have any allergies?

FH
♦ Do any conditions run in your family?
♦ Has anyone in your family had problems during pregnancies?

SH
♦ Do you smoke? Drink alcohol? How much?
♦ Do you take any recreational drugs?
♦ *If answered yes to any of the above* – Have you stopped since you found out you were pregnant? Are you aware of the problems continuing to do so can have on your child?
♦ Who is at home to support you?

Important points
♦ Read the instructions outside the station carefully – does it only ask you to take a history? You may well be required not only to take a history but also to examine the patient, give your diagnosis and determine your investigations and management
♦ Consider at the start whether or not the patient is well enough to take a history from; if the patient is critically unwell, then an ABCDE approach should be initiated ASAP and the history should be sought later
♦ If the patient is haemodynamically stable but you suspect urgent assessment is needed, consider taking a shortened history of the symptoms and then move on to examination and investigations

Differential diagnosis
In many cases, the cause of antepartum haemorrhage is of undetermined origin.

Placenta praevia
♦ Placenta lying in the lower uterine segment; often found incidentally by USS
♦ Intermittent painless bleeding of increasing intensity and frequency
♦ Foetal distress is not common, but can occur with complications of praevia
♦ Risk factors include previous smoking, increasing age and obstetric complications, such as previous praevia, miscarriage and spontaneous abortion

Placental abruption
♦ Placenta either partially or completely detaches from uterus
♦ Painful bleeding with foetal distress
♦ Bleeding may be concealed and therefore not appear as severe as it actually is
♦ Risk factors include smoking, trauma, previous abruption and multiparity

Non-pregnancy-related causes
Cervical ectropion
+ Common in pregnancy
+ Red ring around cervical os on examination with speculum

Cervical polyp
+ Bleeding may occur post-coitally (contact bleeding) or anytime

Cervical cancer
+ Bleeding may occur post-coitally (contact bleeding) or anytime
+ History of multiple partners, STIs, smoking, missed smears, weight loss, loss of appetite

Investigations
+ An ABCDE approach should be used if the patient is acutely unwell (Airways, Breathing, Circulation, Disability and Exposure) – in this case, resuscitating the patient is the primary objective; the patient should be admitted to hospital
+ Bloods – FBC, crossmatch and clotting
+ Must not perform vaginal examination unless placenta praevia excluded by USS, as massive haemorrhage may be provoked
+ Antenatal examination – breech presentation with transverse lie common in praevia
+ Pelvic USS
+ Cardiotocography – evidence of foetal distress? Monitor foetal well-being

Management
+ If required, resuscitation (100% oxygen, large-bore cannulae and fluids)
+ Give analgesia if needed
+ Prophylactic anti-D immunoglobulin for rhesus-negative women
+ Admission until delivery by Caesarean section at 39 weeks or praevia
+ Urgent Caesarean section if foetal distress or severe bleeding

Vaginal discharge
HPC
- **Open question** – Can you tell me about the discharge?
- **Onset** – When did you first notice it?
- **Colour** – What colour is it? Is there any blood?
- **Odour** – Does it have a bad smell?
- **Amount** – How much discharge have you noticed?

Pain
- **Dysuria** – Have you noticed a burning pain when you pass water?
- **Abdo pain** – Have you had any pain in your tummy anywhere recently? *If so, SOCRATES*
- **Dyspareunia** – Have you had any pain during sex? *If so*, where is the pain? Is it a deep pain or a pain on entering?

MenstRUAL history
- How have your periods been recently?
- **Regularity** – How often are your periods? How long do they usually last for?
- **Underwear** – Do you suffer from heavy or painful periods?
- **Age at menarche** – What age were you when you had your first period?
- **Last menstrual period** – When was the first day of your last period?
- **Toxic shock syndrome** – Do you use tampons? Is there any chance you have forgotten to remove a tampon?

Sexual history
Prepare patient for more personal questions, e.g. 'I need to ask some more personal questions now. Is that OK?'
- **Last cervical smear** – When was your last smear? What were the results?
- **Sexually active?** – Are you sexually active?
- **Contraception** – Have you used contraception each time? What method of contraception are you using? (*If the Pill*): Are you remembering to take it regularly? (*If depot used*): When was your last injection? (*If coil used*): When was your coil last checked?
- **Last sexual contact** – Can you tell me when you last had any form of sex?
- **Partner(s)** – Was this with a casual or regular partner? Can I ask if the partner was male or female? How long have you been sleeping with him/her? Where is he/she from? Does he/she have any symptoms or diagnoses?
- **Condoms** – Do you use condoms? All the time?
- **Type of intercourse** – What type of sex do you have? (*vaginal/oral-genital/ genital-oral/genital-anal*)
- **Other sexual contact** – Have you had sex with anybody else in the last 3 months? (*If yes, repeat for each partner*)

ICE
- What do you think is going on? Is there anything you are particularly worried about? Is there anything in particular you would like the doctor to do?

PMH

- Do you suffer from any medical conditions?
- Have you ever had an STI? *If so, specify which one, when, how it was treated and whether the partner(s) was also treated*

DH

- Are you taking any medications?
- Do you have any allergies?

FH

- Do any conditions run in the family?

SH

- Do you drink alcohol? Smoke? How much?
- Do you take any recreational drugs?
- Are you currently working?
- Who is at home?

Important points

- Stress confidentiality aspect to patient
- Non-judgemental approach throughout history is obviously imperative
- Prepare grounds for sexual history before beginning that aspect
- In the sexual history, start with the least intrusive questions and gradually work your way to the potentially most embarrassing ones
- Never take a sexual history in parallel – one partner at a time only
- See patient alone – partners, family or friends may prevent the patient from revealing personal information
- Do not make assumptions about sexual orientation and relationships – use neutral terms such as 'partner'
- Remember STIs 'hunt in packs'. If they have one STI, they may well have another
- Never forget to ask when their last smear was performed – cervical cancer is strongly linked with human papillomavirus infection, which is passed on sexually

Differential diagnosis

Physiological discharge (normal)

- Clear/creamy, thin and stringy discharge
- Amount varies, but typically increases with pregnancy, COCP, around ovulation and during sexual arousal

Sexually transmitted infection

- *Chlamydia trachomatis* – although asymptomatic in the majority of women, chlamydia can cause copious purulent discharge and dysuria
- *Trichomonas vaginalis* – copious amounts of green/yellow discharge that may smell fishy

♦ *Neisseria gonorrhoeae* – often asymptomatic in women, but can cause purulent discharge
♦ HIV, syphilis, genital herpes and genital warts are not associated with vaginal discharge themselves, although as STIs 'hunt in packs', discharge is likely to be present in these cases as well

Non-sexually transmitted infection
♦ Vulvovaginal candidiasis (thrush) – thick, white 'cottage cheese' discharge, with an itchy, red and tender vagina; associated with pregnancy, COCP, antibiotics and immunodeficiency
♦ Bacterial vaginosis – grey-white, fishy-smelling discharge predisposed to by increasing vaginal pH levels (e.g. by sperm, menstruation or using soaps), which kills protective lactobacilli

Pelvic inflammatory disease
♦ Often asymptomatic, presenting later as subfertility or a menstrual disorder
♦ Vaginal discharge, dyspareunia and abnormal vaginal bleeding may occur
♦ History of previously known STIs may not be present, as could be asymptomatic

Foreign body
♦ Most commonly, forgetting to remove a tampon after menstruation
♦ Foul-smelling
♦ Can result in toxic shock syndrome

Genital tract malignancy
♦ Red/brown discharge (blood), likely to be smelly

Investigations
♦ Pelvic examination to look for structural abnormalities, presence of foreign bodies and cervical excitation (for pelvic inflammatory disease)
♦ High vaginal swab for bacterial vaginosis, candida, trichomonas and gonorrhoea (culture)
♦ Endocervical swabs for gonorrhoea (culture) and chlamydia (PCR analysis)
♦ Cervical smear test if not already performed under Cervical Screening Programme
♦ Urgent referral for any patient with suspicion of a genital tract malignancy

Management
♦ Removal of foreign bodies to prevent toxic shock syndrome
♦ Trichomonas and bacterial vaginosis ('fishy'-smelling ones!) – metronidazole
♦ Vulvovaginal candidiasis – clotrimazole pessary or oral fluconazole stat dose
♦ Chlamydia – stat dose of azithromycin or 14-day course of doxycycline
♦ Gonorrhoea – stat dose of oral cefixime or IM ceftriaxone
♦ Pelvic inflammatory disease – analgesia and ceftriaxone IM, followed by a 14-day course of metronidazole and either doxycycline or ofloxacin

Subfertility

In any history regarding a couple's difficulty conceiving, it is extremely important that both of the couple are present and that questions are directed at both of them, as the problem could lie with either one.

General questions (check both partners' responses)
◆ Do you have regular sex? How often?
◆ How long have you been trying for a baby?
◆ Do either of you have any problems having sex? Any pain during sex?
◆ Have you had any previous pregnancies together or with other partners?

ICE
◆ Have you got any ideas yourself why you are struggling to conceive at the moment? I understand this must be very difficult for you, but is there anything in particular you're worried about or would like to discuss?

To the woman

HPC
MenstRUAL history
◆ **Regularity** – How often are your periods? How long do they last for?
◆ **Underwear** – Do you suffer from heavy or painful periods?
◆ **Age at menarche** – How old were you when you had your first period?
◆ **Last menstrual period** – When was the first day of your last period?

Note: If menstrual irregularities are detected, take relevant history of this problem (*see* Amenorrhoea/oligomenorrhoea history, p. 172).

PMH
◆ Have you ever suffered from any medical conditions?
◆ *Ask specifically about miscarriages, polycystic ovarian syndrome, STIs and previous cancer*

DH
◆ Are you currently taking any medications?
◆ Do you have any allergies?
◆ Have you tried taking any medications to assist conception previously?
◆ What contraception have you used in the past? *Take full details*

FH
◆ Has anyone in your family had difficulty in conceiving a child?

SH
◆ Are you currently employed? Does this job involve long periods away from your partner?

- Do you smoke?
- Do you drink alcohol?
- Have you ever taken any recreational drugs?
- I'm sorry, I know this is a personal question, but can I ask how much you weigh?

To the man
PMH
- Have you ever suffered serious trauma to your genitalia?
- Have you ever suffered from any medical conditions?
- Have you ever had a vasectomy?
- *Ask specifically about mumps, STIs, testicular torsion and previous cancer*

DH
- Are you currently taking any medications?

FH
- Has anyone in your family had difficulty in conceiving a child?

SH
- Are you currently employed? Does this job involve long periods away from your partner?
- Do you smoke?
- Do you drink alcohol?
- Have you ever taken any recreational drugs?

Differential diagnosis
The cause of subfertility can be due to problems with the male, female or both. In many couples, the cause is unexplained, of whom many will conceive at a later date.

General causes
- Not having regular satisfactory sexual intercourse
  - Dyspareunia
  - Psychosexual issues
  - Partner away for large periods of time
  - Premature ejaculation before penetration achieved
- Recreational drugs, alcohol and smoking can all impair fertility

Female causes
- Age – female fertility tends to decrease after mid-thirties
- Being overweight
- Systemic conditions, e.g. SLE
- Iatrogenic causes, e.g. pelvic surgery or chemotherapy
- Ovulatory disorders
  - Polycystic ovarian syndrome

- Hyperprolactinaemia
- Thyroid disorders
- Premature menopause
- Hypogonadotrophic hypogonadism
- Tubal pathology
  - Pelvic inflammatory disease
  - Endometriosis
- Uterine pathology
  - Fibroids
  - Uterine abnormalities

Male causes
- Testicular trauma
- Testicular torsion
- Bilateral undescended testicles
- Systemic conditions
- Chemotherapy
- Mumps with orchitis
- Gonorrhoea and chlamydia
- Retrograde ejaculation after transurethral resection of the prostate

Investigations
- Abdominal and bimanual examination
  - Uterine abnormalities
  - Ovarian cysts
  - Cervical excitation for possible pelvic inflammatory disease
  - Vaginismus
  - Painful nodules in pouch of Douglas may indicate endometriosis
- Testicular examination for varicocoeles
- Serum progesterone levels on day 21 of menstrual cycle to assess ovulation
- TFT, prolactin
- Semen analysis may reveal low sperm count or poor motility
- Pelvic USS
- Hysterosalpingogram

Management
- Support and reassurance and advice on need for regular sexual intercourse
- Manage problems with weight, smoking, alcohol and drugs
- Consider psychotherapy for those with psychosexual issues
- Clomiphene to stimulate ovulation in those with oligo-ovulation or anovulation such as polycystic ovarian syndrome
- In vitro fertilisation where there is a problem with the Fallopian tubes or sperm quality
- As a last resort, raise the possibility of adoption if it seems pregnancy is highly unlikely

Urinary incontinence
HPC
Urinary history
- **Onset** – How long has this been going on for?
- **Frequency** – How often do you pass water in a day? More than six times?
- **Nocturia** – How many times do you go during the night? More than twice?
- **Amount** – How much water do you pass each time? *Large or small amounts?*
- **Urge** – Do you ever get the strong urge to go all of a sudden? Have there been times where you haven't been able to make it in time?
- **Stress** – Have you noticed any leaks when straining, coughing or walking?
- **Pads** – Do you use pads to help keep yourself dry? How many do you use in a day? What type of pads do you use? Contipads or nappies?
- **Access** – Do you have easy access to a toilet all the time? Do you always make sure you know where the toilets are when going out?

Urological history (for men)
- **Start** – Do you find that it takes a while to get the stream going?
- **Middle** – When you get going, is the stream weak or strong? Do you have to stop and start several times when passing water?
- **End** – Is there prolonged dribbling at the end? Do you have the feeling that after passing water, there is still some left to pass?

Obstetric history (for women)
- **Prolapse** – Do you have a heavy, dragging sensation down below? Have you noticed anything protruding from there when you cough? *If prolapse suspected, ask the following questions:*
  - **Parity** – How many children do you have? Were they big babies at birth?
  - **Delivery** – Were they delivered normally? Were there any complications?
  - **Menopause** – Have you gone through the change yet?

Other symptoms
- **Open question** – Have you been suffering from any other symptoms?
- **Haematuria** – Have you noticed any blood in your urine?
- **Pain** – Do you get a burning pain when passing water? Have you experienced any pain in your tummy or your sides? *If so, SOCRATES*
- **Fever** – Do you feel ill or feverish?
- **Constipation** – Do you suffer from constipation?
- **Neurological** – Do you have any muscle weakness or disability?
- **Metastatic disease** – Do you have any pains in your bones? Any weight loss?

ICE
- Do you have any idea what might be causing this? How are you coping with this problem? How does this affect you day to day? Is there anything you are particularly worried about or would like to discuss?

PMH

- Do you suffer from any medical conditions?
- *Ask specifically about hypertension, diabetes, multiple sclerosis and Parkinson's disease*

DH

- Are you currently taking any medication?
- *Ask specifically about diuretics ('water tablets')*

FH

- Do any conditions run in the family?
- Has anyone in your family suffered from similar problems? *If so*, what did they have done about it? Is this something you have thought about?

SH

- Do you drink much tea, coffee or fizzy drinks?
- Do you drink anything in the couple of hours before you go to bed?
- Are you still able to go out and meet friends or do you find yourself too restricted by this?
- Do you drink alcohol? Smoke? How much?
- Are you currently working? What did you use to work as?

Important points

- This is often an embarrassing complaint for patients, so use tact and try ways to make the patient feel more comfortable talking to you – tell the patient that one in five people suffer with incontinence, and most for many years before they can talk about it
- Communication skills are very important – it often takes many years for a patient to approach a doctor about incontinence, as they are so embarrassed by the problem
- The psychosocial impact of incontinence is huge – quality of life is reduced, depression and sexual dysfunction are more common and many take time off work due to the problem
- Social history is important – are they drinking lots of caffeine? Fluid before bed?

Differential diagnosis

The aetiology of urinary incontinence is often multifactorial. Broadly speaking, it can be divided into stress incontinence, urge incontinence and mixed incontinence.

Stress incontinence

- Weak/damaged pelvic floor or anal sphincter
- Risk factors – multiparity, complications of vaginal delivery, surgery, perineal tear and episiotomy
- Vaginal prolapse may be seen with symptoms of a heavy, dragging sensation

Urge incontinence
- BPH or prostatic carcinoma
  - Very common in elderly males
  - Urinary symptoms include hesitancy, intermittency, weak stream, terminal dribbling and feeling of incomplete bladder emptying
  - Bone pain, weight loss, jaundice all indicate metastatic carcinoma
- Autonomic neuropathy
  - E.g. diabetes mellitus, multiple sclerosis and Parkinson's disease
  - Other neurological symptoms likely to be present
- Infection
  - Local irritation leads to urinary symptoms
  - Burning pain on micturition, fever, flank/groin/back pain, haematuria, confusion, nausea and vomiting
- Stool impaction

Investigations
- For women:
  - Abdominal examination (palpable bladder)
  - PV examination (structural abnormalities)
  - Urine dipstick and MSU
  - Urodynamic studies
  - Urgent referral if macroscopic haematuria or microscopic haematuria > 50 years old
- For men:
  - Abdominal examination
  - Digital rectal examination (enlarged prostate)
  - Bloods – FBC, LFT, U&E, bone profile (evidence of metastatic disease)
  - PSA
  - Urodynamic studies
  - Urgent transrectal USS and biopsy if hard, irregular prostate or raised age-specific PSA
  - MRI & bone scan if indicated

Management
- Conservative – lifestyle advice (e.g. reduce caffeine intake, no fluids before bed) and pelvic floor exercises
- Medication – duloxetine if surgery contraindicated and conservative measures fail
- Surgery – retropubic midurethral tape, colposuspension and/or sling
- BPH – alpha blockers (e.g. tamsulosin) and 5-alpha reductase inhibitors (e.g. finasteride); transurethral resection of the prostate if medical treatment fails
- Prostatic carcinoma – watchful waiting and surveillance; radical prostatectomy; orchidectomy; hormonal therapy, e.g. goserelin and/or radiotherapy

Amenorrhoea/oligomenorrhoea
HPC
Menstrual history

◆ **Onset** – How long has this been going on for?
◆ **LMP** – When did you have your last period?
◆ **Previous** – What were your periods like before?
◆ **Regularity** – Were they regular? How often did they come?
◆ **Duration** – How long did they last for?
◆ **Age at menarche** – What age were you when you had your first period?

Differential questions

◆ **Pregnancy**
  ● Is there any chance you could be pregnant?
  ● Are you sexually active?
  ● What type of contraception have you been using?
◆ **Polycystic ovarian syndrome**
  ● Are you affected by acne?
  ● Do you find you have lots of hair growing in unusual places like your face, chest or legs?
  ● How has your weight been? Have you struggled to keep it down?
◆ **Thyroid dysfunction**
  ● You mentioned your weight earlier. What has your appetite been like?
  ● Have you noticed a tremor in your hands at all?
  ● Do you find you struggle with either hot or cold temperatures particularly?
  ● How have your bowels been? How regularly do you pass motions?
  ● Have you noticed any changes in your skin or hair?
◆ **Hypogonadotropic hypogonadism**
  ● How often do you exercise? (*per week*)
  ● You talked about your appetite earlier. What do you eat in a typical day?
  ● Have you been feeling low in mood or anxious at all recently?
◆ **Perimenopause/menopause**
  ● Have you been suffering from problems with sweating recently?
  ● Have you experienced any hot flushes?
  ● Has anyone commented on you being tired or irritable at all recently?
  ● Can I ask how your libido has been recently? Have you found sex painful recently?
◆ **Hyperprolactinaemia**
  ● Have you noticed any discharge from your nipples?
  ● Have you had any problems with your vision?

ICE

◆ Do you have any idea yourself what might be going on? Is there anything that you are particularly worried about or would like to discuss?

Obstetric history

+ Do you have any children?
+ Have you previously had any problems trying to conceive? *If so*, do you know why that is?

PMH

+ Do you suffer from any medical conditions?
+ *Ask specifically about thyroid disease, polycystic ovarian syndrome, diabetes and eating disorders*

DH

+ Are you currently taking any medications?
+ Are you on any contraception? Which one? How long have you been taking it? What were your periods like before you started taking it?

FH

+ Do any conditions run in your family?
+ *Ask specifically about autoimmune disease and thyroid disease*
+ Do you know what age your mum was when she reached menopause?

SH

+ Do you smoke? How many cigarettes do you smoke a day? For how long have you smoked?
+ Do you drink alcohol? How much do you drink in a week?

Important points

+ Always consider if the patient could be pregnant
+ What contraception are they currently utilising? Could this affect their menstrual cycle?

Differential diagnosis

Amenorrhoea can either be primary (menses not started by age of 16 years) or secondary (previously normal menses ceased for at least 6 months). Oligomenorrhoea is where the patient experiences menses infrequently, every 35 days to 6 months. This is common in both those who have recently undergone menarche and those who are reaching menopause, but also occurs in several conditions. Depending on the age of the patient, various differentials will be more or less likely.

Primary amenorrhoea

+ Not reached menarche by age 16 years
+ Most commonly constitutional delay; less commonly due to Turner's syndrome, testicular feminisation or polycystic ovarian syndrome
+ In constitutional delay, the patient's mothers and sisters may also have been late in starting

Pregnancy

- Always ask if there is any chance the patient could be pregnant and explore
- Morning sickness, abdominal distension/weight gain, possible implantation bleed 6–12 days after fertilisation, changes in mood

Drug-induced

- Progesterone-only contraception in particular can cause periods to stop
- Reverses within a year upon stopping medication

Polycystic ovarian syndrome

- Symptoms due to excessive amounts of androgenic hormones
- Hirsutism, acne, weight gain, subfertility and polycystic ovaries seen on USS
- Oligomenorrhoea more commonly, but can also present as amenorrhoea
- Insulin resistance and therefore obesity and diabetes associated with condition

Hyperthyroidism

- Intolerance to heat, tremor, weight loss despite increased appetite, frequent bowel movements, protruding eyes, goitre and either oligomenorrhoea or amenorrhoea

Hypothyroidism

- Intolerance to cold, dry coarse skin, weight gain despite poor appetite, constipation, hair thinning, feeling slowed down and menstrual irregularities
- More often causes menorrhagia but can present as irregular periods

Hypogonadotropic hypogonadism

- Low FSH and LH levels
- Most common causes – starvation, excessive exercise, anorexia nervosa, depression, stress, chronic illness and marijuana use

Menopause

- In perimenopausal period ('the change'), symptoms are experienced
- Hot flushes, irregular periods, profuse sweating, irritability, loss of libido, vaginal atrophy
- Menopause occurs when periods have been absent for at least 12 consecutive months
- Premature menopause if onset before 40 years

Hyperprolactinaemia

- Galactorrhoea, amenorrhoea/oligomenorrhoea and subfertility
- Macroprolactinomas may compress optic nerve, leading to bitemporal hemianopia
- Other causes – pregnancy, breastfeeding, stress, drugs, pituitary stalk damage

Investigations

◆ PV examination (assess for vaginal atrophy and ovarian cysts)
◆ Pregnancy test
◆ Bloods – FSH, LH, oestrogen, TFTs and prolactin
◆ Pelvic USS to assess for polycystic ovaries
◆ MRI of head to assess for pituitary and hypothalamic causes

Management

As well as that listed below, also consider the patient's desire for pregnancy. If they are trying to conceive, then offer counselling for the couple for advice. Ovulation-inducing medications may be considered.

◆ Polycystic ovarian syndrome – weight loss and a healthy diet if obese or having difficulty conceiving; COCP can help with hirsutism and regulate periods; metformin for insulin resistance; laparoscopic ovarian drilling
◆ Hyperthyroidism – propranolol and carbimazole initially; radioiodine or surgery where medical treatment fails
◆ Hypothyroidism – thyroxine
◆ Hypogonadotropic hypogonadism – lifestyle advice and CBT if indicated
◆ Menopause – topical lubricant, cream or oestrogen for vaginal atrophy and/or systemic hormone replacement therapy
◆ Hyperprolactinaemia – bromocriptine and surgery if visual defect present

Paediatrics

Paediatric history template 178
Vomiting 180
Failure to thrive 183
Convulsions 187
Developmental delay. 191
Cough 195
Behaviour 198

Paediatric history template

HPC

- *Sequence of events*
- *Symptom analysis*
- *Relevant systems review*

Pregnancy and birth history

- **Prenatal**
  - Any maternal illnesses during pregnancy? (*diabetes, pre-eclampsia, infections*)
  - Did the mother smoke, take alcohol or drugs during pregnancy?
  - Complications during pregnancy and labour
- **Natal**
  - Was it a normal delivery, assisted or Caesarean section?
  - Did the pregnancy reach term? What was his birthweight?
- **Post-natal**
  - Was the child well?
  - Did he require admission?

Feeding history (infants & toddlers)

- Is/was the child bottle-fed or breastfed? *Details of feeding*
- At what age were solids introduced?
- Was there any difficulty weaning the child?

Development history

- Has he met all his developmental milestones so far?
- Has anyone had any concerns about his development?
- *Take full developmental history if appropriate; otherwise check a couple of milestones*
- When did he say his first word?
- When did he start walking unsupported?

Immunisation history

- Is the child up to date with all his vaccinations?
- When was his last one? What was it for?

ICE

- What do you think might be going on? Is there anything you are particularly worried about or would like to discuss?

PMH

- How has the child been before this episode? Any previous illnesses/accidents?

DH

- Does the child take any medications (including inhalers)? Allergies?

FH

- Do any conditions run in the family?
- Check for pattern of inheritance (*draw a family tree if time, or mention it to examiner*)
- Is there any consanguinity?

SH

- Who is at home? Are the parents still together?
- Check how things are at home – Are the parents employed? Alcohol/drug abuse or smoking?
- How is the child in different environments (i.e. school and home)?

Important points

- Always establish first who it is you are talking to – Is it the mother, father, relative, social worker, foster parent or the child?
- Make sure you know the age of the child, as this will shape the rest of the history
- Adapt the history for the child's age and situation, e.g. if they are an adolescent with a cough, a full developmental and feeding history would be inappropriate!

Vomiting

HPC

O'SOCRATES

- **Open question** – Can you describe his vomiting to me?
- **State** child's age
- **Onset** – When did he start vomiting?
- **Character/colour** – What colour is the vomitus? (*blood, bile, milky*)
- **Radiation** – Does it hit the wall? (*projectile/regurgitation/possetting*)
- **Associated symptoms** – *see later*
- **Timing** – How long does the episode last for? Is there any particular time when the vomiting starts? Is there any relation to feeds?
- **Exacerbating factors** – Does anything bring the vomiting on? Is it worse when the child is lying down or sitting up?
- **Subsequently** – How does he feel afterwards? Is he hungry for more food?

Associated symptoms – ILL BUGS

- **ILL** – Has he been ill or irritable? *If so*, when was he last well?
- **Bowels** – What are his stools like? Does he complain of tummy-ache?
- **Urine** – Have you noticed any strange/offensive smell in his urine? Has he complained of any pain?
- **General** – Have you noticed a fever or a rash? Has he seemed drowsy? Is he sleeping well? Is he still wetting his nappies? (*Hydration status*)
- **Scales** – Is he growing normally? Has he been gaining weight?

ICE

- What do you think is causing the vomiting? Is there anything you are particularly concerned about? Are you particularly worried about him?

Feeding history (infants and toddlers)

- What is his appetite like? Is he hungry? Is he fussy about which food he eats?
- What is his feeding pattern like? What does he eat? How often? Where?
- Is he breast- or bottle-fed? If weaned, at what age was he weaned? Any problems related to particular kinds of food like milk?

Pregnancy and birth history

- **Prenatal** – Were there any problems during pregnancy or labour?
- **Perinatal** – Did the pregnancy reach term? What was his birthweight?
- **Post-natal** – Was he well after delivery?

Development history

- Has he met all of his milestones so far?
- Has anyone had any concerns about his development?
- *Check a couple of milestones appropriate for the child's age*

Immunisation history

- Is he up to date with all his jabs?

PMH

- How has he been before this episode? Any previous illnesses?

DH

- Has he been given any medications?
- Does he have any allergies that you are aware of? (*E.g. lactose*)

FH

- Do any conditions run in the family?
- *Ask specifically about coeliac disease and IBD*

SH

- Who is at home? Are you still with his mother/father? Does he have any siblings?
- Is the child at school, playgroup or nursery?
- Has anyone at home or at school had similar symptoms?

Important points

- The age of the child is very important in this case, as some conditions are more common in certain age groups
- It is always important to check the relationship between the adult and child and to make sure that the adult you are speaking to is the legal guardian or has parental responsibility of the child
- Remember to quantify the feeds; vomiting may simply be due to overfeeding of the child!
- Always remember to rule out more serious conditions such as meningitis

Differential diagnosis

Gastro-oesophageal reflux disease

- Very common in first year of life due to functional immaturity of lower oesophageal sphincter
- Recurrent regurgitation and vomiting related to feeds; relieved by sitting up
- Child can be distressed after feeding – feeding and behavioural difficulties
- Other risk factors include premature delivery and cerebral palsy

Pyloric stenosis

- Peak age 2–7 weeks
- Projectile vomiting straight after feed
- Child remains hungry after vomiting
- Complications: dehydration, constipation and failure to thrive

Intussusception

- Peak age 5–10 months

- Paroxysms of colicky abdominal pain around every 10–20 minutes; often indicated by child drawing knees into their chest and inconsolable crying
- Early – vomiting which rapidly becomes bile-stained
- Later – mucus and blood per rectum (redcurrant jelly stools)

Coeliac disease
- Peak age 9 months–3 years (typically after weaning)
- Vomiting, pallor, steatorrhoea, abdominal distension and failure to thrive

Meningitis
- Vomiting – will not take feeds
- Fever, irritable or lethargic
- Non-blanching purpuric rash
- Cold extremities
- Signs of increased intracranial pressure, i.e. bulging fontanelle

Gastroenteritis
- Diarrhoea and vomiting
- Fever, irritable and unwell
- History of recent travel
- There may well be someone in family or school with similar symptoms

Investigations
- Physical examination of child – if satisfied from history and examination it is GORD or uncomplicated gastroenteritis, no further investigations are required
- U&Es (to look for any signs of dehydration)
- Pyloric stenosis – test-feed, feeling for olive-shaped mass in epigastrium and looking for visible peristalsis; USS to confirm
- Intussusception – USS abdomen and barium enema
- Coeliac disease – antiendomysial and antigliadin autoantibodies; duodenal biopsy to confirm
- Meningitis – neuro exam and look for rash, lumbar puncture (CT head first if possible raised intracranial pressure), blood cultures and blood glucose

Management
- Rehydration – with oral intake if mild–moderate; IV fluids if severe
- Rehydration is usually all that is required in GORD and gastroenteritis
- Pyloric stenosis – pyloromyotomy
- Intussusception – air enema/barium enema if diagnosed early, otherwise surgery
- Coeliac disease – lifelong gluten-free diet
- Meningitis – antibiotics (e.g. benzylpenicillin IM initially and cefotaxime IV) in bacterial meningitis; antipyretics and analgesia in viral meningitis

Failure to thrive
PC
+ 'My child isn't growing/putting on weight like other kids his age'

HPC
Growth timeline
+ **Clarify** – Are you concerned about his height, weight or both?
+ **Onset** – When did you first notice this?
+ **Progression** – Has he always been a small child? What was his birthweight? How has his growth been since birth? Has he been putting any weight/height on? Has he lost any weight?

Other symptoms
+ **Illness** – Has he been ill or irritable? Has he been an ill child since birth?
+ **Infection** – Has he had any recent or recurrent infections?
+ **Nappies** – How many wet and dirty nappies does he produce in a day?
+ **Stools** – Can I ask what his stools look like? Has he had any diarrhoea?
+ **Vomiting** – Has he been vomiting at all?
+ **Abdominal pain** – Any tummy-ache?
+ **Cough** – Has he had a cough? *If so*, for how long? Does he bring anything up?

ICE
+ Have you got any ideas yourself what might be going on? What is your biggest concern? How is this affecting them? Is he being bullied at school?

Feeding history
+ Can you tell me about his feeding routine?
+ What does he eat? Is he fussy about which food he eats?
+ What is his appetite like? How often does he eat? Where does he eat?
+ Was he breast- or bottle-fed? What age was he weaned at? Were there any difficulties weaning him?
+ *If still being bottle-/breastfed* – Are you having any difficulties with his feeds?

Pregnancy and birth history
+ **Prenatal**
  - Did you/the mother have any significant illnesses during pregnancy?
  - Did you/the mother smoke, take alcohol or drugs during pregnancy?
  - Were there any complications during pregnancy or labour?
+ **Perinatal**
  - Did the pregnancy reach term?
  - Was it a normal delivery?
+ **Post-natal**
  - Was he well at birth?
  - Did he pass his first stool at the right time?

Development history
+ Has he met all of his developmental milestones so far?
+ Has anyone had any concerns about his development?
+ *Take full developmental history if appropriate; otherwise check a couple of milestones appropriate for their age*
+ When did he say his first word?
+ When did he start walking unsupported?

Immunisation history
+ Is he up to date with all his jabs?

PMH
+ Does he have any medical or genetic problems you know of?

DH
+ Has he been given any medications?
+ Does he have any allergies?

FH
+ Do any conditions run in the family?
+ *Ask specifically about coeliac disease, cystic fibrosis and diabetes*
+ How were you and your partner growing up? Did you have any problems?

SH
+ Who is at home? Does he have any siblings? How are they?
+ How are things at home? Do you feel you have enough support?
+ Is he at school, playgroup or nursery? How is he doing there?

Important points
+ The age of the child is very important in this case, as feeding patterns, amount and products are different at different ages
+ It is always important to check the relationship between the adult and child and to make sure that the adult you are speaking to is the legal guardian or has parental responsibility of the child
+ Note how the parent speaks about the child – Are they caring and concerned or cold and distant? This could help to determine whether the child is at risk
+ Substitute 'your child' with child's actual name

Differential diagnosis
Organic causes
Prenatal
+ Prematurity, maternal malnutrition, congenital infections, intrauterine growth restriction and toxin exposure in utero (e.g. alcohol [foetal alcoholic syndrome], cigarettes or recreational drugs)

Intake issues
- Inability to suck or swallow in neuromuscular disorders (e.g. cerebral palsy)
- Cleft palate, long-standing GORD or vomiting after feeds

Malabsorption
- Diarrhoea will be a prominent feature – note when this occurs
- Cystic fibrosis – cough with sputum, URTI
- Coeliac disease (typically as solids are introduced), IBD, cow's-milk intolerance and unspecified chronic diarrhoea can also cause malabsorption

Metabolic disorders
- Poor metabolism in hypothyroidism and diabetes
- Increased metabolic demand in hyperthyroidism, heart and renal failure

Non-organic causes
Constitutional delay
- Genetic predisposition (i.e. short parents, short child!)
- No other problems identified in history

Inadequate feeds
- Not being fed enough or often enough
- Distractions at mealtime
- Poor breastfeeding technique
- Bottle feeds not made up correctly
- Could be due to lack of knowledge/supervision or child neglect
- Contributing factors include lack of support and problems in home environment

Investigations
- Physical examination, including cardiac (murmurs), respiratory (wheeze, crepitations), abdominal (masses) and neurological (cranial nerves and limbs)
- Plot measurements on growth and weight centile charts
- If an obvious cause is identified, no further tests may be required
- Blood tests – FBC, U&Es, ESR, TFTs, LFTs, glucose
- Urinalysis and urine culture
- Stool culture for ova/parasites/cysts and faecal fat for malabsorption
- Antigliadin and antiendomysial autoantibodies for coeliac disease
- Sweat test for cystic fibrosis

Management
- General measures
  - Provide a suitable feeding environment
  - Parent education on feeding requirements, breastfeeding technique, etc.

◆ A multidisciplinary approach may be required
  ● Health visitors may help if the parents are not coping well at home
  ● Dieticians provide invaluable input – particularly in coeliac disease
  ● Paediatricians for assessment and management of organic conditions
  ● Where child neglect is suspected, social services should be involved

Convulsions

HPC

♦ Did you witness the episode? Can you talk me through exactly what happened?

♦ Where did it occur? When did it occur?

Before

♦ **Precipitating factors** – What was he doing before it started?
  - Was he playing video games or watching television?
  - Was he unwell? Did he have a fever? If so, how high? Did you give him anything for this? Did he have a rash?
  - Was he tired?
  - Was he scared or crying immediately before the episode?
  - Had he fallen and hit his head any time before the episode?

♦ **Aura** – Did he describe any funny feelings or sensations before the episode?

During

♦ **Duration** – How long did the episode last for?

♦ **LOC** – Did he lose consciousness at any point? Did he fall to the floor? If so, did he hit his head?

♦ **Jerks** – Was he shaking? *If so*, can you describe it please? Did his whole body jerk or only part of it?

♦ **Tongue-biting** – Did he bite his tongue? *If so*, the front or the side of his tongue?

♦ **Incontinence** – Did he pass water or soil himself?

♦ **Pallor/cyanosis** – Did he appear pale or blue during the episode?

After

♦ **Post-ictal state** – How did he feel immediately after the episode? Does he remember the event?

♦ **Previous episodes** – Has this ever happened before?

♦ **General health** – How is he doing generally? Is he growing and gaining weight normally? Is he sleeping well?

ICE

♦ What do you think caused the episode? Is there anything you are particularly concerned about? How do you feel after witnessing the episode?

Pregnancy and birth history

♦ **Prenatal**
  - Did you/the mother have any illnesses during pregnancy?
  - Did you/the mother smoke, drink alcohol or take recreational drugs in pregnancy?
  - Were there any complications during pregnancy or labour?

◆ **Perinatal**
  ● Was it a normal delivery, assisted or Caesarean section?
  ● Did the pregnancy reach term? What was his birthweight?
◆ **Post-natal**
  ● Was he well after delivery?
  ● Did he require admission?

Development history

◆ Has he met all of his developmental milestones so far?
◆ Has anyone had any concerns about his development?
◆ *Take full developmental history if appropriate; otherwise check a couple of milestones appropriate for their age*
◆ When did he say his first word?
◆ When did he start walking unsupported?

Immunisation history

◆ Is he up to date with all his jabs?

Feeding history (infants and toddlers)

◆ What is his appetite like?
◆ What is he eating at the moment? How often does he eat?
◆ At what age was he weaned? Any problems?

PMH

◆ Does he have any other medical problems?
◆ *Ask specifically about cerebral palsy, tuberous sclerosis and previous meningitis*

DH

◆ Is he on any medication at the moment?
◆ Does he have any allergies?

FH

◆ Do any conditions run in the family?
◆ *Ask specifically about a family history of epilepsy and febrile convulsions*

SH

◆ Who is at home? Are there any problems at home? Does he have any siblings?
◆ Is he at school, playgroup or nursery? How are things there?

Important points

◆ It is always important to check the relationship between the adult and child and to make sure that the adult you are speaking to is the legal guardian or has parental responsibility of the child
◆ The pregnancy and birth history is very important here, as any injuries or toxins during this time could have predisposed the child to having convulsions

♦ The parent is likely to be very distressed and concerned in this history, as it is distressing for anyone to witness their child convulsing – an empathetic and understanding nature is imperative

♦ Commonly, the parent's primary concern is that their child has epilepsy – often it is the child's first seizure and there is a clear history of fever, so it is acceptable to explain that he is likely suffering from febrile convulsions (explain what this means and measures the parents can take to prevent re-occurrences) and that a diagnosis of epilepsy cannot be made on the basis of one seizure alone in any case

Differential diagnosis

Febrile convulsions
♦ Affects children between the ages of 6 months and 5 years
♦ High temperature (> 38°C) at time of seizure, usually due to a common viral infection
♦ Tonic and/or clonic, symmetrical, generalised seizure usually lasting < 5 minutes
♦ No signs of central nervous system infection, focal neurological signs or a previous history of epilepsy

Reflex anoxic seizure
♦ Brief and spontaneous, paroxysmal episodes triggered by fear, anxiety or pain
♦ Episode lasts < 1 minute
♦ Typically, the child suddenly becomes pale and limp, losing consciousness briefly
♦ This is then followed by involuntary tonic and/or clonic movements of the limbs
♦ Urinary incontinence may be evident, and the child may feel groggy afterwards
♦ Unlike in epilepsy, tongue-biting is not a feature

Breath-holding attack
♦ Often precipitated by emotion such as anger or frustration or trauma
♦ A crying episode often ensues, breath is withheld and pallor or cyanosis develop
♦ Loss of consciousness may occur, but recovery is usually quick

Epilepsy
♦ Risk factors include birth asphyxia, cerebral palsy and trauma
♦ Watching television and lack of sleep are known precipitants
♦ Partial seizures cause symptoms depending on the part of the cerebrum affected, e.g. strange sensations, déjà vu, paraesthesia down one limb; lasts up to a few minutes
  ● Simple – no loss of consciousness
  ● Complex – impaired level of consciousness

- Generalised seizures involve the entire cerebrum
  - Absence – frequent episodes where the child stops what he is doing, remains still and stares vacantly for 2–3 seconds
  - Tonic–clonic – classic episodes of stiffening of the body lasting for 10–20 seconds, followed by violent shaking of limbs; tongue-biting, incontinence and post-ictal state are associated with this type; can last up to 2–3 minutes
- There are many other variants associated with childhood epilepsy

Meningitis
- Unwell and drowsy child prior to convulsions with pyrexia
- Non-blanching rash of meningococcal septicaemia may be present

Others
- Tuberous sclerosis – condition which causes multiple non-cancerous tumours to develop around the body, including the brain
- Vasovagal syncope
- Benign paroxysmal vertigo
- Hypoglycaemic attack

Investigations
- Neurological examination (including Kernig's sign, Brudzinski's sign and looking for bulging fontanelle) and inspection for any rashes
- If normal examination, including observations, and typical history of febrile convulsions, no further investigations may be required
- Lumbar puncture and blood cultures if there is any suspicion of meningitis
- Blood tests – FBC, U&Es, LFTs, glucose (hypoglycaemia)
- ECG to rule out underlying arrhythmias
- EEG – best done during a seizure

Treatment
- Parent education
- Put child in the recovery position when convulsing and call for help
- Keep temperature down when pyrexial, and give plenty of fluids and paracetamol
- Usually for reflex anoxic seizures and breath-holding attacks, parent reassurance is all that is required
- Epilepsy
  - Not everyone requires treatment
  - Specialist paediatric or neurological referral is required
  - Generally, sodium valproate is reserved for those with partial seizures and carbamazepine for those with generalised seizures

Developmental delay

HPC

◆ How old is your child? (*Consider now whether the child is truly late in meeting the milestone*)

Developmental history

◆ How has your child been developing otherwise? I know he can't walk at the moment, but what can he do? Do you have his red book with you?
◆ Are you particularly concerned about his development?
◆ Do you know what age *his parents* first started walking at? Siblings? What age were they?
◆ OK, I want to ask you a list of quick questions to assess your child's development. Is that OK?

Gross motor

◆ Does he favour either hand? How long has he been like that for?
◆ What age did your child first hold his head up? Sit up? Crawl?
◆ How does he crawl? On both knees? With one leg trailing behind? Bottom-shuffling?

Vision and fine motor

◆ When did you notice he first started following things with his eyes? Reaching for things? Transferring things from one hand to the other? Make a pincer grip?

Hearing, speech and language

◆ Does he react or turn to sounds that are out of sight?
◆ What age did he first use babble? What can he say now?

Social, emotional and behavioural

◆ What age did you first see him smile? Wave bye-bye?
◆ Does he pretend play with teddy? Play with others? (NB: these milestones are typically met past 18 months of age)
◆ Is he otherwise well at the moment?

Pregnancy and birth history

◆ How was the pregnancy? Did you/the mother have any illnesses during it?
◆ Did you/the mother smoke, drink alcohol or take any drugs whilst pregnant?
◆ Did the pregnancy reach term? How was the childbirth? Was it a normal delivery?
◆ Did he have any problems soon after childbirth? Did he need resuscitation?

Immunisation history

◆ Is he up to date with all his jabs?

Feeding history
+ Did he feed well from the start?
+ Does he cope OK with solid foods?

ICE
+ Is there anything you think might be going on or are worried about?

PMH
+ Has he had any serious illnesses?
+ *Ask specifically about meningitis*

DH
+ Is he taking any medications? Allergies?

FH
+ Do any conditions run in the family?
+ *Ask specifically about Duchenne's muscular atrophy*

SH
+ Who's at home?
+ Does he get the chance to move around?
+ Is he at preschool or play group? How is he doing there?

TABLE 1 Developmental milestones and their limit ages

Gross motor		Vision and fine motor		Hearing, speech and language		Social, emotional and behavioural	
Milestone	*Limit age (months)*	*Milestone*	*Limit age (months)*	*Milestone*	*Limit age (months)*	*Milestone*	*Limit age (months)*
Holding head up	4	Fixing eyes and following visually	2	Turning to sounds	4	Smiling	2
Sitting unsupported	9	Reaching for objects	6	Babble	8	Waves bye-bye	10
Standing independently	12	Transferring between hands	8	First word	15	Feeds self	18
Walking independently	18	Using pincer grip	12	Talking in sentences	36	Symbolic play	30

Important points
+ Presenting complaint could be anything regarding developmental delay, but the principles are the same and, in any case, a *full* developmental history is required

♦ A child should NOT favour either hand in the first year of life, as hand dominance is not acquired until 1–2 years old – this implies pathology is present, e.g. cerebral palsy
♦ Smiling socially by 2 months old is a consistent milestone, whereas crawling is an inconsistent milestone
♦ Up to six words by 2 years old is the minimum acceptable

Differential diagnosis

The differential for developmental delay is very large, depending on which of the four fields of development are affected. If all four fields are affected, it implies a global developmental delay. If one field is affected significantly more than the others, there is a specific developmental delay. Differential diagnosis for two of the commonest presentations of developmental delay is considered below.

Delay in motor development
Normal variation
♦ Often a family history of delayed development of motor skills
♦ Normal in all other aspects, but slow in developing motor skills
♦ When motor skills are achieved, they are of a normal standard
♦ Children who are bottom-shufflers or commando crawlers are more likely to develop walking skills later than children who crawl on their knees and hands

Cerebral palsy
♦ Disorder of motor function caused by non-progressive pathology to the developing brain
♦ Abnormal tone and posture and delayed achievement of motor milestones
♦ Often widespread dysfunction, e.g. learning difficulties and epilepsy
♦ Three types: spastic, ataxic hypotonic and dyskinetic cerebral palsy
♦ Causes (usually in antenatal period):
  ● Antenatal – vascular occlusion, congenital infection, maldevelopment of the brain
  ● Perinatal – prolonged hypoxia in birth
  ● Post-natal – head trauma, meningoencephalitis, periventricular leukomalacia
♦ Premature babies are at an increased risk of developing periventricular leukomalacia

Duchenne's muscular dystrophy
♦ X-linked recessive condition (affects boys only)
♦ Delayed achievement of motor milestones; waddling gait and possible global delay
♦ Gower's sign: child uses hands to 'climb up' legs in order to stand up

Other
♦ Causes of global developmental delay – e.g. Down syndrome, tuberous sclerosis

- Metabolic disorder – e.g. rickets, hypoglycaemia
- Environmental – e.g. a child who is always kept in the cot or bedridden through illness

Delay in speech and language development
Normal variation
- Often a family history of delayed speech development
- Otherwise normal and appropriately developing child

Hearing difficulties
- Otitis media with effusion is common in childhood and can cause delayed speech and language development and later affect performance in school

Autistic spectrum disorder
- Impaired reciprocal social interaction and communication and repetitive stereotyped behaviours
- Delayed or complete lack of speech development with no other forms of communication, such as miming or gesturing, attempted in its place
- Abnormal social, emotional and behavioural development – e.g. playing in isolation

Other
- Cleft palate
- Learning difficulties
- Environmental deprivation and neglect

Investigations
- Observation of child at play
- Neurological examination
- Ear examination and hearing assessment for speech and language delay
- Creatinine phosphokinase levels (Duchenne's muscular dystrophy)
- Chromosomal karyotyping

Management
- MDT approach involving physiotherapists, paediatricians, audiologists, psychologists, social workers, speech and language therapists and occupational therapists
- Treat underlying condition where possible (e.g. otitis media, rickets, hypoglycaemia)

Cough
HPC
Timeline
- **Onset** – How long has it been going on for? When was he last well?
- **Timing** – Is it there all the time? Is it worse at any particular time of the day? Does it vary with the seasons or weather?
- **Triggers** – Does anything set the cough off? Has he put anything up his nose or in his mouth? Does anyone at home smoke?
- **Character** – Can you describe the cough? Is it barking? Wet? Whoop sound?

Associated features
- **Discharge** – Any discharge from his nose? What colour is it? Is it smelly?
- **Sputum** – Does he cough anything up? *If so*, how much? What colour is it?
- **Wheeze** – Have you noticed a wheeze or any other strange sounds?
- **URTI** – Does he currently have a headache, runny nose, sore throat or painful ears? Anyone in the family or at school with similar symptoms?
- **Breathlessness** – Has he been breathless? *If so, quantify exercise tolerance*
- **Chest pain** – Does he have any chest pain? *If so, SOCRATES*
- **Growth** – Is he growing well? Has he lost any weight?

ICE
- What do you think is causing this? What is your biggest concern? Are you worried about anything else? How has this affected him?

Feeding history (infants and toddlers)
- What is his appetite like?
- Does he choke or gag at all when eating solids?

Pregnancy and birth history
- **Prenatal** – Were there any problems during pregnancy or labour? Did you/his mother smoke during pregnancy?
- **Perinatal** – Did the pregnancy reach term? What was his birthweight?
- **Post-natal** – Were there any problems after delivery? Did he pass his first stool at the right time? (*Meconium ileus*)

Development history
- Has he met all his developmental milestones so far?
- Has anyone had any concerns about his development?
- *Take full developmental history if appropriate; otherwise check a couple of milestones appropriate for their age, e.g.*
  - When did he say his first word?
  - When did he start walking unsupported?

Immunisation history
- Is he up to date with all his jabs?

PMH
- How was he before this episode?
- *Ask specifically about eczema, hay fever and previous infections (quantify)*

DH
- Does he take any medications or inhalers?
- Does he have any allergies?

FH
- Do any conditions run in the family?
- *Ask specifically about asthma, hay fever, eczema and cystic fibrosis*

SH
- Who is at home? Any pets? *If so,* how long have you had the pet?
- What is the housing like?
- Does anyone smoke at home?
- Is he at school, playgroup or nursery? Does he have any hobbies?

Important points
- It is always important to check the relationship between the adult and child and to make sure that the adult you are speaking to is the legal guardian or has parental responsibility of the child
- The description of the cough is very important, as it could distinguish what the diagnosis is from quite early on
- Finding out whether there are any pets at home or any allergies that the child has is also very useful

Differential diagnosis
Asthma
- Dry cough with diurnal variation, wheeze and breathlessness/chest tightness
- Responds well to bronchodilators
- Family history and personal history of atopy
- Precipitated by cold weather, exercise, pets and cigarette smoke

Cystic fibrosis
- Productive cough, wheeze and repeated respiratory infections
- Failure to thrive, with meconium ileus (neonate), diarrhoea and steatorrhoea due to malabsorption
- Autosomal recessive condition

Bronchiolitis
- Common viral illness seen in the first year of life
- Raspy cough, wheeze, coryzal symptoms and fever
- Less wet nappies, poor feeding and grunting sounds indicate severe infection

Pertussis
- Sore throat, dry cough and coryzal symptoms in early phase
- Intense bouts of coughing for 1–2 mins with characteristic whoop sound when trying to breathe in between coughs
- Episodes of going red or blue in the face and vomiting after bouts may occur
- Can take up to 3 months before stopping

Croup
- Viral illness causing a barking cough with stridor and coryzal symptoms
- Commonest in first few years of life and usually self-limiting
- Can cause airway obstruction, however, which must be taken seriously

Epiglottitis
- Fever, drooling, dysphagia, dysphonia, soft stridor and a severe sore throat
- Most commonly seen in children 1–8 years old
- Very unwell, with rapidly increasing dyspnoea and airway obstruction

Others
- Foreign body – sudden onset of coughing and stridor or nasal discharge
- URTI – general coryzal symptoms
- Tonsillitis – sore throat and fever
- Otitis media – may have otalgia, or be seen to pull on their ear
- Pneumonia – productive cough, fever, unwell with grunting sounds

Investigations
- Physical examination, including full ENT and respiratory examination
- Pernasal swab for pertussis
- Throat swab if necessary
- Nasopharyngeal mucus secretion analysis (in bronchiolitis)
- Peak flow if asthma suspected and child is capable (usually > 7 years old)
- Sweat test if cystic fibrosis is suspected
- Fibre-optic laryngoscopy in theatre for patients with suspected epiglottitis

Management
- Most URTIs are self-limiting, therefore parental advice – monitor their temperature and give paracetamol and plenty of fluids
- Avoidance of allergens or trigger factors in asthma, plus inhalers in a stepwise approach – salbutamol PRN, then add a regular corticosteroid, then add a regular long-acting beta2-agonist, then consider a leukotriene antagonist
- Antibiotics may be considered for more serious infections and for those with cystic fibrosis (who need specialist multidisciplinary care)
- Epiglottitis – involve senior paediatrician and anaesthetist straight away; start a broad-spectrum antibiotic such as cefotaxime; likely to need intubation

Behaviour

PC

1. 'I'm finding it hard to cope with my child's behaviour; he never listens to me'
2. 'The school has complained about my child's behaviour'

HPC

- Tell me about what has happened regarding your child
- How would you describe his behaviour?
- Has he always been this way? When did you first notice it?
- Can you think of anything that may have triggered this behaviour?

Environments

- **Home** – How is he at home? Who else it at home? What are his relationships like with them?
- **School** – How is he at school? Is it a mainstream school? What do the teachers say about him? How is he doing academically?
- How is he elsewhere? Can you take him out to public places like restaurants?

Conduct

- Does he get into trouble often? If conduct is an issue, explore in more detail:
  - **Disobedience** – Does he respect any rules or authority?
  - **Truancy** – Has he ever missed school?
  - **Bullying** – Does he get involved in bullying?
  - **Violence** – Can he be violent or cruel to either humans or animals?
  - **Law** – Has he ever been in trouble with the law? *If so*, what for?
  - **Substances** – Has he ever drunk alcohol, smoked or used illicit drugs?

Attention deficit hyperactivity disorder features

- **Hyperactivity** – Would you say he is hyperactive? Is he restless, fidgety and constantly talking? Does he 'bounce off the walls'?
- **Impulsiveness** – Does he take turns or constantly interrupt conversations?
- **Inattention** – How are his concentration levels? Is he easily distracted?

Autistic features

- **Communication** – Does he have any difficulties with communication?
- **Social impairment** – Does he have friends? Is he able to play with other children? Does he enjoy imaginary play?
- **Repetitive behaviours** – Does he like to follow a strict routine? *If so*, what would happen if this was changed?

ICE

- What do you think is going on? What is your main concern?

Pregnancy and birth history
+ **Prenatal** – Were there any problems during pregnancy or labour?
+ **Perinatal** – Did the pregnancy reach term? What was his birthweight?
+ **Post-natal** – Were there any problems after delivery?

Development history
+ Did he meet all of his developmental milestones at the correct times?
+ Has anyone shown any concern regarding his development?
+ *Take full developmental history if appropriate* (e.g. *delay in speech/language*)
+ When did you first see him smile?
+ When did he say his first word?
+ Does he respond when you call his name? Have you got any concerns about his hearing?

Immunisation history
+ Is he up to date with all his jabs?

PMH
+ Does he suffer with any known behavioural conditions or learning difficulties?

DH
+ Is he on any medications at the moment?
+ Does he have any allergies you know of?

FH
+ Does anybody in the family have behaviour problems or learning difficulties?

SH
+ How are things at home? Are there any problems? What are his siblings like?
+ Has anyone at home ever been in trouble with the law?

Important points
+ It is always important to check the relationship between the adult and child and to make sure that the adult you are speaking to is the legal guardian or has parental responsibility of the child
+ You must rule out hearing difficulties as a cause of 'not listening'
+ Always assess whether the features are evident across different environments

Differential diagnosis
Attention deficit hyperactivity disorder
+ Usually affects children between the age of 3 and 7 years
+ Inattention – short attention span with difficulty concentrating in class
+ Hyperactivity – unable to sit still for long periods and constantly fidgeting
+ Impulsiveness – unable to wait in turn and little sense of danger
+ Symptoms must be present for > 6 months across at least two environments

Conduct disorder

+ Usually affects children and adolescents above the age of 7 years
+ Violence, bullying, theft, vandalism and cruelty to animals
+ Problems at school, including truancy and often expulsion
+ Disobedience and lack of respect for authority
+ Can be precipitated by situation at home, including being bullied or abused, parental drug or alcohol addiction, family conflicts or big changes at home

Autistic spectrum disorder

+ Social impairment – lack of interest in playing with others/imaginary play
+ Communication impairment – delayed language development, few social gestures
+ Repetitive behaviours – deviating from set routines causes great difficulty to them; stereotypy is another feature (e.g. making particular sounds)
+ Risk factors: gestational age < 35 weeks, family history, chromosomal disorders, cerebral palsy

Other differentials

+ Oppositional defiant disorder – less severe variant of conduct disorder
+ Hearing or visual impairment – evidence of developmental delay
+ Learning difficulties
+ Tic disorder, e.g. Tourette's syndrome

Investigations

+ Physical examination is required to rule out any medical causes
+ Hearing assessment including audiometry if a concern is identified
+ Speech and language assessment if developmentally delayed
+ Multidisciplinary approach observing the child in different settings

Management

+ A multidisciplinary approach is vital, involving the child, parents, paediatricians, general practitioners, psychologists, speech and language therapists, teachers, special education needs coordinators and others
+ Autistic spectrum disorder – behavioural modification, speech and language therapy, occupational therapy and the Treatment and Education of Autistic and Communication-related handicapped CHildren (TEACHH) method are just some of many possible management strategies
+ ADHD – behavioural modification, parent education and family therapy; methylphenidate can be considered in moderate–severe cases of ADHD
+ Conduct disorder – behavioural modification and family therapy

Musculoskeletal medicine

Back pain. 202
Joint pain 206

Back pain

HPC

O'SOCRATES

- **Open question** – Tell me about the pain
- **Site** – Where exactly do you feel the pain? Can you point to the area?
- **Onset** – When did you first notice the pain? Did it come on suddenly or gradually? Was there any history of trauma? Have you had it before? *If so*, is it the same pain or different?
- **Character** – What is the pain like?
- **Radiation** – Does the pain go anywhere else? Does it travel down your legs? If so, how far?
- **Associated features** – *see later*
- **Timing** – Is the pain always there or does it come and go? Is it worse at any particular time of the day?
- **Exacerbating/relieving factors** – Does anything make the pain better? Anything make it worse? Is it made better or worse by movement? Is it made better or worse by rest? Is it worse when lying down or standing? Is it tender when you press on it? Have you tried taking any painkillers for it?
- **Severity** – If you had to score the pain between 1 and 10, with 10 being the worst pain you can imagine, how would you score your pain?

Associated features

- **Cord compression** – Have you had any problems with your waterworks? Bowels? Have your legs been feeling weaker than usual? Have you had any strange sensations down your legs or buttocks? *Men only!* – Have you had any difficulty in gaining an erection?
- **Inflammatory** – Is your back stiff in the morning? *If so*, how long does that last for?
- **Constitutional** – Have you noticed any significant weight loss over the past few months? How is your appetite? Have you been feeling feverish or ill recently? How has your mood been?

ICE

- What do you think is wrong? What is your biggest concern?

PMH

- Do you suffer from any medical conditions?
- *Ask specifically about osteoporosis, arthritis, TB and previous cancer*
- Have you ever suffered from back pain before?

DH

- Are you currently taking any medications?
- What have you tried for the pain in the past?
- Do you have any allergies?

FH

+ Do any conditions run in the family?
+ *Ask specifically about ankylosing spondylitis and osteoporosis*
+ Has anyone in your family ever been troubled by back pain?

SH

+ Are you currently employed? If yes, what do you do? What effect has this had on your job?
+ Do you smoke? How many do you smoke a day? For how many years?
+ Do you drink alcohol? How much do you drink in a week?
+ Do you use any recreational drugs?
+ Do you cope at home? Who is at home with you?

Important points

+ Always enquire about red-flag symptoms to rule out sinister causes
+ Cord compression and cauda equina are medical emergencies and must be sought after in the history

TABLE 2 Red-flag and yellow-flag symptoms for back pain

Red-flag symptoms (indicative of serious pathology)	Yellow-flag symptoms (prognostic of long-term disability)
Progressively worsening pain that is not relieved by rest	Negative attitude that their back pain is severely disabling
Age of onset < 20 or > 50 years	Belief that activity is harmful to recovery
Urinary/faecal incontinence, leg weakness, saddle anaesthesia	Belief that passive treatment will be beneficial
History of cancer; weight loss; fever	Depression and social withdrawal
Severe trauma or minor trauma in the presence of known osteoporosis	Financial difficulties

Differential diagnosis

Mechanical lower-back pain (including lumbar spondylosis)

+ Usually a localised pain that worsens with movement and changes in posture
+ There may be a history of trauma/heavy lifting or it could be spontaneous
+ There will frequently be a history of previous similar episodes over a number of years
+ No features of systemic illness, nor neurological symptoms

Prolapsed intervertebral disc

+ Sudden severe lower-back pain often brought on by heavy lifting
+ Nerve-root involvement (most commonly sciatic nerve) classically causes a shooting pain down the leg that extends below the knee, with paraesthesia in a dermatomal pattern

Malignancy
+ Systemically unwell (e.g. weight loss) and symptoms from primary malignancy
+ Usually of gradual onset, with constant pain not relieved by rest
+ History of malignancy with tendency to metastasise to bone, such as multiple myeloma, prostatic or breast carcinoma

Cauda equina syndrome
+ Urinary and faecal incontinence
+ Sensory numbness of buttocks and backs of thighs and weakness of legs
+ The most common causes are malignancy and infection

Osteoporotic crush fracture
+ Risk factors for osteoporosis include increasing age, female sex, corticosteroid therapy, premature menopause (< 40 years), smoking and malabsorption
+ Sudden localised back pain after minimal trauma – sometimes a sneeze is all it needs

Seronegative spondyloarthropathy (HLA-B27–associated conditions)
+ Ankylosing spondylitis, psoriatic arthritis, enteropathic arthritis and reactive arthritis
+ Typically a young male of Caucasian origin
+ Morning back stiffness lasting > 1 hour which improves with exercise
+ Reduced range of movement of spine, with characteristic question mark posture in the late stages

Infection
+ Severe back pain in a systemically unwell patient with fever and night sweats
+ Past history of TB may suggest Pott's disease

Spinal canal stenosis
+ Associated with degenerative changes, so more common in an elderly population
+ Pain brought on by exercise and relieved by rest
+ Patient usually feels more comfortable in a slightly stooped forward position

Non-spinal causes of back pain
+ Dissecting aortic aneurysm – sudden-onset severe 'tearing' back pain typically felt between the shoulder blades
+ Fibromyalgia – more generalised aches and pains, including arthralgia and myalgia
+ Pancreatitis, endometriosis and renal calculi are rare causes of back pain

Investigations
+ Back examination and lower-limb neurological examination
+ Bloods – FBC, LFTs, U&Es, CRP and ESR
+ Chest X-ray and QuantiFERON-TB Gold if TB suspected

+ MRI (not needed if the history suggests uncomplicated mechanical back pain)
+ Urgent MRI/CT scan if cord compression or cauda equina is suspected
+ X-ray and a subsequent DEXA scan if a crush fracture is suspected

Management
+ Simple back pain (including prolapsed intervertebral disc):
  - Advise to stay active and avoid prolonged bed rest
  - Physiotherapy, regular analgesia and consider short-course muscle relaxants
+ Serious pathology or red-flag symptoms:
  - Cord compression – dexamethasone and urgent surgery; radiotherapy in malignancy
  - Cauda equina syndrome – urgent surgery
  - Ankylosing spondylitis – NSAIDs
  - Osteoporosis – bisphosphonates, vitamin D and calcium supplements

Joint pain

HPC

O'SOCRATES

- **Open question** – Can you tell me about the pain?
- **Site** – Where is the pain?
- **Onset** – When did you first notice the pain? Was there any history of trauma?
- **Character** – What does the pain feel like?
- **Radiation** – Do you have pain anywhere else? (other joints)
- **Associated features** – *see later*
- **Timing** – When do you get the pain? Is it there all the time or does it come and go? Are the symptoms worse at any particular time of the day?
- **Exacerbating/relieving factors** – Does anything make it better? Does anything make it worse? Is it made better or worse by the cold? Is it made better or worse by exercise? Does resting the joint help the symptoms at all? What painkillers have you tried so far? Do they help?
- **Severity** – If you had to rate the pain from 1 to 10, with 10 being the worst pain you can imagine, how would you score your pain? How do your symptoms affect your day-to-day life? Is there anything you find you cannot do now as a result of your symptoms?

Associated features

- **Stiffness** – Have you noticed any stiffness in your joint(s) when you wake up in the morning? How long does that last for?
- **Swelling** – Have you noticed any swelling, redness or heat in your joint(s)?

Extra-articular features

- Other than the pain and swelling, how have you been otherwise?
- **Infections** – Have you had any recent infections?
- **Rashes** – Have you noticed any rashes anywhere on your body?
- **Enteropathy** – Have you had any diarrhoea?
- **Uveitis/iritis** – Have you had painful or red eyes?
- **Spondyloarthropathy** – Have you had any back pain? Do you get any stiffness in your back in the morning, and if so, for how long?
- **CTD** – Do you suffer from mouth ulcers? Dry eyes or mouth? Painfully cold hands that change colour?

ICE

- What do you think is wrong? What is your biggest concern?

PMH

- Do you suffer from any medical conditions?
- *Ask specifically about psoriasis, IBD, STIs, conjunctivitis and uveitis*
- Have you ever suffered from problems with your joint(s) in the past?

DH

+ Do you take any medications?
+ *Ask specifically about thiazides (could precipitate gout)*

FH

+ Do any conditions run in your family?
+ *Ask specifically about arthritis and clarify what kind of arthritis*

SH

+ Do you smoke? How many cigarettes do you smoke a day? For how long have you smoked?
+ Do you drink alcohol? How much do you drink in a week?
+ Are you currently employed? If so, what do you work as? How have your problems affected your job?
+ What is your current home situation? How are you coping at home?

Important points

+ Exercise, swelling and heat improving stiffness are important features that indicate an inflammatory cause
+ Many arthritides are associated with systemic symptoms – extra-articular features may provide useful clues as to the underlying pathology
+ It is very important to ascertain a timeline of the patient's symptoms – for diagnosis of chronic conditions like RA, the symptoms must be present for at least 6 weeks, whereas an acutely swollen joint is likely to have an entirely different diagnosis
+ Beware of the acutely hot, swollen joint – could it be septic arthritis?

Differential diagnosis

Is it a definite history of arthritis? Is it inflammatory or non-inflammatory? Redness, heat, swelling and early morning stiffness for more than 1 hour suggest inflammatory arthritis. What is the pattern of joints involved? Is it small or large; symmetrical or asymmetrical; mono-, oligo- or polyarthritis?

Inflammatory conditions
Rheumatoid arthritis

+ Symmetrical polyarthritis that typically causes synovitis in small joints – particularly the hands and feet – although large joints can also be affected
+ Morning stiffness lasting > 1 hour, along with pain that improves with exercise

Seronegative spondyloarthropathy (HLA-B27-associated conditions)

+ Psoriatic arthritis, ankylosing spondylitis, enteropathic arthritis and reactive arthritis
+ Typically, there is an asymmetrical oligoarthritis affecting large joints – the spine is frequently involved with sacroiliitis most commonly – and enthesitis
+ Morning stiffness lasting > 1 hour, along with pain that improves with exercise
+ Particularly consider in a history of psoriasis/bowel disorders/recent infection

Systemic lupus erythematosus
+ Arthralgia and/or symmetrical small-joint polyarthritis (non-erosive)
+ Typically affects non-Caucasian females, with age of onset in early adulthood
+ Common features include oral ulcers, Raynaud's phenomenon, dry eyes and/
  or mouth, photosensitivity, malar rash, discoid rash, fever and general malaise

Non-inflammatory conditions
Osteoarthritis
+ Pain in older patients that is worse with exercise and at least partially relieved
  by rest
+ Symmetrical oligo- or polyarthritis that most frequently affects hips, knees
  and hands
+ History of previous injury to the joint and/or obesity (especially for knee OA)

Gout
+ Joint pain, oedema and erythema that develops acutely (classically overnight)
+ Usually it is a large-joint monoarthritis affecting the first metatarsophalangeal
  joint, but it can affect any joint and can be polyarticular
+ History of excessive alcohol and red-meat consumption, hypertension, renal
  failure, diuretics and being male!

Fibromyalgia
+ Myalgia that can be reproduced over specific trigger points without joint
  involvement
+ Patient may complain of swelling despite objectively no swelling being present
+ Associated with depression and irritable bowel syndrome

Septic arthritis
+ An acutely hot, very painful and swollen joint in an unwell patient with fever
+ There may be a history of immunosuppression
+ Trauma
+ Unilateral swollen joint with local tenderness and preceding history of injury

Investigations
+ Examine joint(s) in question and screen other joints; look for evidence of
  extra-articular features such as rash, nail changes, gouty tophi, lung fibrosis
+ Bloods – FBC, U&Es, LFTs, CRP and ESR
+ Autoimmune screen if suspecting RA or CTD
+ Blood cultures if suspecting septic arthritis
+ Serum urate if suspecting gout
+ Acute setting: joint aspiration and synovial fluid analysis for septic arthritis
  and gout
+ X-rays of joint(s) for evidence of erosive disease (usually of hands and feet)
+ Chest X-ray if possibility of interstitial lung disease

Management

- Physiotherapy has a role in each chronic condition
- Osteoarthritis – exercise, weight loss, regular analgesia and monitoring
- Rheumatoid arthritis – early DMARDs (e.g. methotrexate); anti-TNF therapy if conventional DMARDs fail
- Gout – treat acute attack with NSAIDs; after acute episode resolves, review precipitating factors and consider allopurinol for long-term prevention
- Seronegative spondyloarthropathy – NSAIDs, DMARDs in peripheral arthritis, and anti-TNF therapy
- Lupus – hydroxychloroquine for mild symptoms; steroids and DMARDs for joint disease; high-dose steroids and potent immunosuppressants for end-organ disease
- Fibromyalgia – patient education; amitriptyline currently first-line medication
- Septic arthritis – broad-spectrum IV antibiotics

Ophthalmology

Painful red eye 212
Loss of vision/blurry vision 216

Painful red eye

HPC

O'SOCRATES

- **Open question** – Can you tell me more about the pain?
- **Site** – Is it affecting both eyes or just one? The whole eye or just part of it?
- **Onset** – When did you first notice your eye was red and painful? How did it start? Was is sudden or did it gradually worsen?
- **Character** – Can you describe the pain? Is it a dull ache? Sharp? Irritating?
- **Radiation** – Do you feel the pain anywhere else? Do you get a headache with this pain? *If so, describe*
- **Associated symptoms** – *see later*
- **Timing** – Is the pain always there or does it come and go? *If intermittent,* how long does it last for? How often do you get the pain?
- **Exacerbating/relieving factors** – Is the pain worse on moving your eyes or looking at bright lights? Can you recall any trauma to your eye or foreign object going into your eye?
- **Severity** – How bad is the pain on a scale of 1–10?

Other important eye symptoms

- **Vision** – Is your vision affected? *If so,* in what way? Is it blurry? Are you still able to read small print?
- **Discharge** – Has there been any discharge?
- **Pruritis** – Does your eye itch?
- **Xerophthalmia** – Do you have trouble with dryness?
- **Haloes** – Do you see haloes around bright lights?

Systemic enquiry

- **Fever** – Have you had a fever or been feeling poorly recently?
- **GI** – Do you have any trouble with your bowels? Abdominal pain? Any vomiting?
- **Respiratory** – Have you recently had a bad cough?
- **GUM** – Any urinary symptoms, such as burning when passing urine or discharge? Have you been treated for any STIs?
- **Arthralgia** – Any pain in any joints?
- **Rashes** – Do you have any rashes?

ICE

- What do you think is wrong? Is there anything you are particularly worried about or would like to discuss?

PMH

- Have you ever had any trouble with your eyes in the past?
- Do you wear glasses or have a refractive error? *Long-sighted people are at an increased risk of angle-closure glaucoma*
- *Ask specifically about rheumatoid arthritis, IBD and ankylosing spondylitis*

(HLA-B27–positive patients have a significant risk of anterior uveitis and scleritis)

DH
+ Do you take any medications?
+ *Ask specifically about systemic/topical steroids and topical eye drops*
+ Do you have any allergies? *Allergic conjunctivitis occurs in people who suffer with atopy such as hay fever*

FH
+ Does anyone in the family suffer with eye problems, both recent and old?

SH
+ What do you do for a living? *Is there a high risk of a foreign body? (E.g. blacksmiths classically, engineers or manual labourers)*
+ Do you wear contact lenses? *(Poor contact lens hygiene can cause microbial keratitis)*

Important points
+ A red eye may be obvious, but eye pain can be misleading – if pain is the only symptom, you may need to think laterally, e.g. could this be a cluster headache or other non-ophthalmological issue with referred pain? Similarly, patients may present with what is thought to be a headache or subarachnoid haemorrhage, only to have their red eye neglected
+ Red flags to look out for include visual loss/impairment, a history of trauma or foreign object and the possibility of a chemical injury
+ Although the acute red eye is a common complaint and often entirely benign, it can also represent an acute ocular emergency which requires rapid evaluation and treatment in order to preserve vision – it is therefore important to be able to identify the serious diagnoses so that the appropriate action can be taken if needed to prevent permanent damage to vision

Differential diagnosis
Conjunctivitis (viral, bacterial, allergic)
+ Usually unilateral, but later may become bilateral due to autoinoculation
+ Conjunctival injection (red sclera), watery or purulent discharge
+ Allergic – abrupt onset after exposure, bilateral, with chemosis, pruritis and eyelid oedema; watery discharge with foreign-body sensation, nasal congestion and hives may also be present; tends to have seasonal variation

Acute angle-closure glaucoma
+ Ophthalmological emergency – if not treated rapidly, will result in irreversible damage to the optic disc and retina from pressure-induced ischaemia
+ Presents unilaterally, commonly in the evening due to low light levels causing a mid-dilated pupil, increasing risk of angle closure

♦ Symptoms include red eye, pain (globe, headache and abdominal), blurred vision, haloes around lights and nausea and vomiting

Infectious keratitis (bacterial, fungal, parasitic, herpes simplex, herpes zoster)
♦ Unilaterally painful eye that mimics conjunctivitis
♦ There is a foreign-body sensation, photophobia and reduced vision
♦ Bacterial keratitis is much more likely in contact lens wearers or the immunocompromised
♦ Potentially blinding due to corneal scarring and neovascularisation or perforation – therefore warrants immediate ophthalmological referral

Acute anterior uveitis
♦ Acute pain, often a recurring event, in one eye with associated photophobia, redness and blurred vision
♦ Typically the pain is felt more deeply than in conjunctivitis
♦ *Photophobia occurs because the iris is inflamed, and so miosis is painful*
♦ There may be a background history of HLA-B27-associated spondyloarthropathies, IBD, Reiter's syndrome and/or psoriasis

Episcleritis
♦ Injection of a localised area overlying the sclera with a non-tender globe
♦ Often recurrent and characterised by rapid onset of a dull ache, redness and tenderness

Scleritis
♦ Severely painful, subacute onset with associated tearing and photophobia
♦ Often recurrent and bilateral, though not simultaneously
♦ Strongly associated with rheumatoid arthritis, ANCA-positive vasculitis, SLE and IBD
♦ Potentially sight-threatening, may result in astigmatism

Subconjunctival haemorrhage
♦ Diffusely red eye unilaterally, with no associated pain or visual disturbance
♦ Often after an episode of coughing, vomiting or straining
♦ May be caused by trauma – exclude globe damage or foreign body
♦ Resolves spontaneously

Investigations
♦ Thorough eye examination, including visual fields
♦ Dilated ophthalmoscopy, ideally a slit-lamp examination (do not dilate if you suspect angle closure)
♦ Tonometry
♦ Conjunctival and corneal swabs for culture/PCR
♦ Syphilis serology, chest X-ray and HLA-B27 testing for complex uveitis
♦ Gonioscopy

Management

- Acute angle closure – IV acetazolamide, dexamethasone, pilocarpine, timolol and iopidine, all immediately; peripheral iridotomy
- Viral conjunctivitis – cool compress for symptomatic relief
- Bacterial conjunctivitis – topical chloramphenicol
- Allergic conjunctivitis – topical mast cell stabilisers for prophylaxis; topical antihistamines for symptomatic relief; oral steroids for severe disease
- Herpes simplex keratitis – topical acyclovir
- Herpes zoster ophthalmicus – oral acyclovir
- Anterior uveitis – cycloplegia for symptomatic relief; topical steroid to induce remission

Loss of vision/blurry vision

HPC

- ◆ **Clarify** – What do you mean by loss of vision? Is your vision blurry or are you missing parts of your vision? *If blurry*, do you see double or is it just all unclear? *If double vision*, are the images side by side or one above the other?
- ◆ **Site** – Is this in both eyes or one side only? Is it in the entire eye or part of it? Which part of your vision is missing/affected? Left or right? Upper or lower vision? Do you have tunnel vision?
- ◆ **Onset** – When did you first notice this? How suddenly did it come on? Was it gradual or sudden? Was it like a curtain coming down?
- ◆ **Timing** – How has it changed since you first noticed it? Does it come and go?
- ◆ **Central vision** – Is the centre of your vision affected when you look directly at something?
- ◆ **Colour vision** – Have you noticed a change in your colour vision?
- ◆ **Remaining vision** – How much vision remains? Are you able to recognise faces, read small text or see any light?
- ◆ **Triggers** – Did anything precipitate this? Any history of trauma?

Associated features

- ◆ **Pain** – Do you have any pain in your eyes or around your eyes? Is it painful to move your eyes? Any headache?
- ◆ **Injection** – Have you noticed any redness in your eyes recently?
- ◆ **Flashes and floaters** – Have you noticed any flashes of light or floaters?
- ◆ **Neuro** – Have you seen any zigzag lines? Do you have any weakness or pins and needles? Have you had any trouble with your speech?
- ◆ **Hypertension** – Do you get any morning headaches on waking?
- ◆ **Temporal arteritis** – Do you get a cramping pain in your jaw when chewing food? Is it painful to comb your hair?

ICE

- ◆ What do you think is wrong? Is there anything you are particularly worried about or would like to discuss?

PMH

- ◆ Do you suffer from any medical conditions?
- ◆ *Ask specifically about diabetes, hypertension, atrial fibrillation, IHD, and peripheral vascular disease*
- ◆ Have you ever had any trouble with your eyes in the past? Do you suffer from short-sightedness? Do you see an ophthalmologist regularly or for screening?

DH

- ◆ Have you recently started taking any new medications?
- ◆ *Ask specifically about digoxin*
- ◆ Do you have any allergies?

FH

- Do any conditions run in the family?
- Does anyone in the family have trouble with their vision?
- *Ask specifically about glaucoma and retinitis pigmentosa*

SH

- Do you smoke?
- Do you drink alcohol? Do you drink home-made alcohol?
- Do you take any illicit drugs or inject yourself?
- What is your occupation?
- Do you drive?

Important points

- Beware patients with homonymous defects may report monocular blindness when they mean one side of their visual field is missing
- Similarly, some patients fail to notice a monocular blindness until their good eye is covered
- An instant change in vision is more likely to be due to vascular occlusion
- A horizontal defect suggests a retinal vascular cause; a vertical defect suggests a neuro-ophthalmic problem
- Some drugs have been known to cause sudden disturbance in vision. For example, digoxin can cause the vision to become more yellowish
- IV drug abuse may result in septic emboli in the retinal vessels
- Moonshine and antifreeze have been known to cause toxic optic neuropathy, whilst B_{12} deficiency in alcoholism can result in optic atrophy
- Very important that the patient's ability to drive is approached. It is the patient's responsibility to inform the DVLA

Differential diagnosis

Acute visual loss

Retinal artery occlusion

- Sudden onset of persistent monocular visual loss
- Exact field defect dependent on whether it is a central or branch occlusion (branch occlusion will produce a horizontal field loss)
- Amaurosis fugax, hypercoagulable state and atherosclerotic risk factors may be present

Retinal vein occlusion

- Acute painless monocular mild–moderate visual loss

Temporal arteritis

- May present as a recent severe headache over the temporal region
- Jaw claudication, scalp tenderness and proximal muscle stiffness and aching
- Transient/permanent visual loss, blurred vision and amaurosis fugax
- Patients > 55 years, and if left untreated, will affect the other eye in weeks

Optic neuritis

+ Often young female patients, and may be first presentation of multiple sclerosis
+ Deep pain associated with eye movements and a central scotoma
+ Symptoms exacerbated by raising body temperature (e.g. exercise/hot baths)
+ Neurological symptoms such as weakness or paraesthesia

Retinal detachment

+ Signs and symptoms include flashes of light, floaters and a peripheral scotoma
+ Risk factors include myopia (thin retina), recent cataract surgery and diabetes

Vitreous detachment

+ Common cause of acute visual disturbance, affecting the middle-aged/elderly
+ Chronic floaters, with a sudden increase in the number of floaters and possibly flashing lights as the vitreous starts to pull away from the retina
+ May result in retinal detatchment or vitreal haemorrhage
+ Visual acuity not affected and usually self-limiting

Vitreal haemorrhage

+ Spontaneous bleeding from the retinal vessels into the vitreous
+ Sudden onset of altered vision, blobs and floaters
+ Visual acuity is variable depending on site and size of haemorrhage

Cerebral vascular accident

+ Sudden onset of homonymous visual field defect
+ Patient may describe it as losing vision in one eye when in fact it is the entire left or right visual field that has gone
+ Weakness, paraesthesia, dysphasia and ataxia may also be present

Gradual visual loss
Glaucoma

+ Usually asymptomatic; may develop visual field loss with negative scotomas typically found in the nasal field
+ Blurring and haloes around lights may occur due to corneal oedema
+ Risk factors include Afro-Caribbean ethnicity, diabetes, advanced age, myopia and family history

Cataract

+ History of blurred vision, glare from bright lights, increasing myopia, yellowish/brown discolouration, monocular diplopia and poor night vision
+ Gradual worsening of symptoms
+ Risk factors include advancing age and diabetes

Macular degeneration
+ Gradual onset of worsening visual acuity and a central scotoma
+ Metamorphopsia, where images become distorted, is also a common complaint

Retinitis pigmentosa
+ Nyctalopia, decreased visual acuity and loss of peripheral vision
+ Nearly 50% is inherited in autosomal dominant, recessive or X-linked pattern

Investigations
+ Eye examination including visual fields, acuity and ophthalmoscopy
+ ESR and temporal artery biopsy if suspecting temporal arteritis
+ Ocular coherence topography
+ Fundus fluorescein angiography to help demonstrate macular oedema
+ USS of posterior segment
+ Tonometry and pachymetry where glaucoma is suspected
+ Kinetic perimetry to assess visual fields and glaucoma progression
+ Carotid Doppler and echocardiogram for source of emboli
+ MRI for diagnosis of multiple sclerosis

Management
+ Retinal artery occlusion – ocular massage may help improve outcome
+ Retinal vein occlusion – lifestyle factors (smoking cessation, blood pressure control and diabetic control); ischaemic retinal vein occlusion – panretinal photocoagulation and anti-VEGF antibodies
+ Temporal arteritis – high-dose oral steroids
+ Optic neuritis – IV and oral steroids can hasten recovery of optic neuritis but not improve final vision
+ Retinal detachment – surgical repair
+ Macular degeneration (wet) – intravitreal anti-VEGF therapy
+ Retinitis pigmentosa – vitamin A to slow progression
+ Cataracts – phacoemulsification and implantation of a prosthetic lens

Index

References to tables are in **bold**.

5-alpha reductase inhibitors 95, 98, 171

ABCDE approach
  and antepartum haemorrhage 161–2
  and breathlessness 58
  and haematemesis 76
  and headache 109
  tips for 11
abdominal pain
  acute and chronic 36–7
  in children 182–3
  and diabetes 96–8
  differential diagnosis for 35–6
  and dysuria 92, 94
  and fever 22
  in gynaecological history 154
  history taking for 34–5
  key areas for **36**
  and rectal bleeding 84
  and red eye 212, 214
  and vaginal bleeding 156, 159
  and vaginal discharge 163
abdominal swellings 38, 44, 80, 84, 89
abortion, spontaneous 159, 161
acamprosate 146
ACE inhibitors 55, 59, 63–5, 91, 113
achalasia 72–3
acne 172, 174
acoustic neuroma 119–20, 123
ACS (acute coronary syndrome) 35–6, 53, 55, 57–9, 72
active problem list 5
acyclovir 27, 120, 215
adenosine 62
ADHD (attention deficit hyperactivity disorder) 198–200
affect 2, 5
agoraphobia 131
ALARMS symptoms 71–6
alcohol
  and anxiety 130
  and depression 127
  and dizziness 119–20
  and forgetfulness 137–8

  and gout 208
  and haematemesis 75–6
  and hallucinations 134–5
  and hearing loss 122–4
  and mania 141–2
  and palpitations 61–2
  in pregnancy 183, 187, 191
  and self-harm 150–2
  and subfertility 167–8
  and visual loss 217
alcohol abuse 30, 145
alcohol history 29, 44–5, 144–5
alcohol withdrawal 132, 135
alcoholism
  diagnosis of 145–6
  and fever 21
  and haematemesis 76–7
  and TB 68
  and tiredness 17
  and visual loss 217
alpha blockers 95, 98, 171
Alzheimer's disease 137–8
amenorrhoea 94, 147–9, 166, 172–5
amitriptyline 79, 209
amnesia 103
anaemia
  and bowel habit 78–9
  and depression 127
  and dysphagia 71
  investigations for 19
  management of 19
  and tiredness 16–17
anal fissures 79, 83, 85
analgesics, and headache 109
anaphylaxis 22, 26
angina 52–4, 130–1
angiodysplasia 84–5
angiography 49, 55, 76
angiotensin receptor blockers 65
anhedonia 18, 126–7, 134–5
ankylosing spondylitis 203–5, 207, 212
anorectal disease 79–80, 84
anorexia nervosa 43, 148, 174
antibiotics
  and arthritis 209
  and bruising 29

  and candidiasis 165
  and cough 197
  and fever 23
  and hearing loss 122, 124
  and meningitis 182
  and pneumonia 59, 65, 68
  and rash 27
antidepressants 102, 143, 151
antidiarrhoeals 79, 82
antiemetics 120, 124
antihypertensives 4, 104
antiphospholipid syndrome 160
antipsychotics 135, 142
anxiety
  and alcohol 144
  and bowel habit 80
  and breathlessness 56
  and depression 126–7
  differential diagnosis of 130–2
  and forgetfulness 136
  and hallucinations 133
  history taking for 129–30
  and mania 140, 142
  and numbness 114, 116
  and palpitations 60, 62
  and weight loss 41
aortic aneurysm 36–7, 40, 204
aortic dissection 54–5
aortic stenosis 104–5
aortoenteric fistula 76
appendicitis 35
appetite
  and abdominal pain 34
  and alcohol 144
  and bowel habit 78
  and breathlessness 56
  and bruising 28
  and chest pain 52
  in children 180, 183, 188, 195
  and cough 63
  and depression 126–7, 129, 132
  and dizziness 118
  and fever 20
  and haematemesis 74, 76
  and haematuria 88
  and haemoptysis 66
  and hearing loss 121

221

appetite (*continued*)
and jaundice 44
and lumps 38
and mania 140
and numbness 114
and palpitations 61
and polyuria 96
and rash 24
and rectal bleeding 82
and tiredness 16, 18
and vaginal bleeding 157
and weakness 110
and weight loss 41
appetite suppressants 148
arrhythmias
and claudication 48
and convulsions 190
and falls 102, 104
and palpitations 61
arteriovenous malformations 76
arthralgia 22, 28, 204, 208, 212
arthritis
and back pain 202
and dysuria 93
and falls 104
and fever 21
inflammatory 20, 207
and joint pain 207
and rashes 24
reactive 94, 204, 207
asbestos 57, 63, 67
aspirin
and bruising 28–9
and claudication 47, 49
and haematemesis 74
and stroke 117
asthma 25, 56–8, 63–5, 196–7
ataxia 108, 115, 137, 218
atherosclerosis 5, 48
atrial fibrillation 61–2, 71, 130–1,
146, 216
aura 102–3, 107, 120, 187
autistic spectrum disorders 194,
198, 200
autoimmune disorders
and amenorrhoea 173
and fever 21
and jaundice 45
and tiredness 18
and weakness 111
autoimmune screen 23, 112, 208
azithromycin 94, 165

back pain 202–5
barotrauma 121
Barrett's oesophagus 72
benzodiazepines 62, 135, 142
beta blockers
and anxiety 132
and breathlessness 59
and chest pain 55
and depression 127
and palpitations 62
and tiredness 18

betahistine, prophylactic 120, 124
binge-drinking 44, 141, 146
binge-eating 147, 149
bipolar disorder 126, 128, 135,
140, 142
birth asphyxia 189
bisphosphonates 75, 77, 99, 205
blackouts 110, 114, 118
bladder, hyperactive 97
bladder cancer 89–90
bleeding disorders
and antepartum haemorrhage
160
and haematemesis 74
and haematuria 89
and haemoptysis 66
and headache 107
and rashes 24
and vaginal bleeding 157–8
blindness 109
bloating 78–80
blood pressure
and claudication 49
medications for 47
body language 2
Boerhaave's syndrome 76
bone pain 171
bowel habit
differential diagnosis of 79–80
history taking for 78–9
and malignancy 20
management of 81
and rectal bleeding 83
and tiredness 16
BOWELS mnemonic 78
BPH (benign prostatic
hyperplasia) 88, 90, 94–5, 97–8,
171
BPPV (benign paroxysmal
positional vertigo) 119–20, 190
brain tumour 138
breast cancer 19, 204
breastfeeding 174, 185
breath, shortness of, *see* shortness
of breath
breathlessness
and bronchiectasis 68
and cancer 18
and chest pain 52–4
and cough 64–5
differential diagnosis of 57–8
and haemoptysis 66
history taking for 56–7
management of 58–9
progressive 58, 64, 67
bronchiectasis 64–5, 68
bronchiolitis 196–7
bronchitis, acute 67
bronchodilators 59, 65, 196
bronchoscopy 19, 65, 68
bruising
differential diagnosis of 29–30
and haemoptysis 67
history taking for 28–9

and malignancy 20, 22
management of 30–1
bulbar palsy 71
bulimia nervosa 149
bullying 198, 200

cachexia 22, 41, 79–80, 83–4
Caesarean section 160, 162, 178,
188
caffeine
and dizziness 119–20
and hearing loss 123–4
and incontinence 170
and migraine 107
and palpitation 61–2
CAGE questionnaire 44, 115,
144–5
calcium channel blockers 62,
73, 91
Calgary–Cambridge model, key
elements of 1–3
cancer
and DVT 48
and fever 21
and haemoptysis 66
investigations for 19
and tiredness 16–18
candidiasis 165
CANDITIME surgical sieve 42
cannabis 134–5, 142, 174
cardiac death, sudden 61
cardiac pain 53
cardiovascular disease 145
carotid massage 62
carpal tunnel syndrome 116–17
cataracts 218–19
categorisation, explicit 3
CATS PAWS mnemonic 82
cauda equina 203–5
CBT (cognitive behavioural
therapy)
and alcoholism 146
and amenorrhoea 175
and anxiety 132
and depression 128
and mania 142
and palpitations 62
and tiredness 19
cefotaxime 109, 182, 197
ceftriaxone 94, 165
cellulitis 26–7
cerebral palsy 181, 185, 188–9,
193, 200
cerebral vascular accident 54, 218
cervical cancer 157–8, 162, 164
cervical ectropion 158, 162
cervical spondylosis 112, 116
chairlifts 47, 103, 105
chemotherapy
and cough 65
and fever 23
and haematuria 90
and haemoptysis 68
and hearing loss 122

and ototoxicity 119
and subfertility 167–8
chest, examining 9
chest discomfort 58, 64, 67
chest infection
  and bronchiectasis 68
  recurrent 58, 64, 67
chest pain
  and abdominal pain 34
  and anxiety 129, 131
  and breathlessness 56
  in children 195
  differential diagnosis of 53–4
  and dysphagia 70, 72
  and falls 102, 104
  and haemoptysis 66
  history taking for 52–3
  investigations for 55
  pleuritic 22, 53–4, 57, 64,
    67–8
chest trauma 54, 57
chest X-ray
  and back pain 204
  and breathlessness 58
  and chest pain 55
  and cough 65
  and dysphagia 72
  and fever 23
  and haemoptysis 68
  and lung disease 19, 208
  and psychiatric conditions 135,
    138, 142
  and weakness 112
  and weight loss 43
child neglect 185–6
children
  behavioural problems of
    198–9
  non-accidental injury in 29–30
chlamydia 94, 164–5, 168
chlordiazepoxide 146
chloroquines 119, 122
cholesteatoma 123–4
chronic fatigue syndrome 17–19
chronological approach 15
chunks 3
cirrhosis 46
clarification 2, 4, 8–9
claudication 33, 47–9, 109
cleft palate 185, 194
clomiphene 168
clopidogrel 28, 55, 59
closed questions 2–3, 21, 25
closure 4–6
CLOTS mnemonic 88
clotting disorders 52, 54, 57, 66
cluster headache 107–9, 213
CMV (cytomegalovirus) 43
COCP (combined oral
  contraceptive pill) 158, 164–5,
  175
codeine 79, 82
coeliac disease 80, 84, 181–2,
  184–6

COF RESUS mnemonic 56
colonoscopy 19, 23, 81
colorectal cancer 19, 80, 83–4
colour vision 216
communication skills 11, 17, 127,
  130, 170
condoms 157, 163
conduct disorder 200
conjunctivitis 93–4, 206, 213–15
constipation
  and abdominal pain 35
  factors causing 79
  history taking for 78–9
  and hypercalcaemia 98
  and hypothyroidism 18, 128
  and incontinence 169
  and pyloric stenosis 181
  and rectal bleeding 82
contraception
  and amenorrhoea 172, 174
  and haemoptysis 66
  and migraine 107
  and subfertility 166
  and vaginal bleeding 157
  and vaginal discharge 163
convulsions 187–90
COPD (chronic obstructive
  pulmonary disorder)
  and breathlessness 56–9
  and chest pain 54
  and cough 63–5
  and weight loss 43
corrosives 70
corticosteroids 65, 110, 197, 204
costochondritis 53–4
cough
  and breathlessness 56
  and cancer 16
  and chest pain 52
  in children 64, 183, 185, 195–7
  chronic 58, 64–5
  differential diagnosis for 64–5
  and falls 104
  and haemoptysis 66–8
  history taking for 63–4
  and lumps 38
  and red eye 214
  and URTI 20, 24
  and weight loss 41
Creutzfeldt–Jakob disease 138
Crigler–Najjar syndrome 45
Crohn's disease 36, 79, 81, 85
cross-checking 4
croup 197
CTD (connective tissue disorder)
  20, 22, 43, 206, 208
cues 2, 4–5, 11
CURB-65 score 59, 65, 68
Cushing's syndrome 58, 64, 67
cyanosis 187, 189
cycloplegia 215
cystic fibrosis
  and bronchiectasis 65, 68
  and cough 196–7

and failure to thrive 184–5
and weight loss 42
cystitis 90–1, 93–4, 97–8

deafness
  adult onset 121
  progressive 119, 123
decision making, shared 4
dehydration 127, 181–2
delirium 90, 93, 97, 135, 138
delirium tremens 132, 135, 142,
  146
delusions 128, 133–5, 142
dementia 137–9
demyelinating disorder 115
depression
  and alcohol 144
  and amenorrhoea 174
  differential diagnosis of 127–8
  and fibromyalgia 208
  history taking for 126–7
  and incontinence 170
  management of 19
  and other psychiatric problems
    133, 135–6, 141–2, 150
  and thyroxine 16
  and tiredness 18
  and weight loss 41, 43
depressive pseudodementia 138
dermatitis 25–7
dermatomyositis 67, 111
developmental delay 191–4, 200
developmental milestones **192**
diabetes
  and abdominal pain 35
  and alcohol 145
  and amenorrhoea 174
  and antepartum haemorrhage
    160
  and anxiety 130
  and breathlessness 56
  and chest pain 52–3
  and claudication 47–8
  during pregnancy 178
  and failure to thrive 184–5
  and fever 21
  and haematuria 88
  and incontinence 170
  management of 19
  and numbness 114
  and polyuria 96–7
  and stroke 71
  and tiredness 16–18
  and visual loss 216, 218
  and weakness 110
diabetes insipidus 98
diabetes mellitus 18, 97–8, 171
diabetic ketoacidosis 97–8
diarrhoea
  and anxiety 132
  bloody 30, 80–1, 84–5
  chronic 80, 84, 185
  and cystic fibrosis 196
  and dysuria 92

diarrhoea (*continued*)
   and failure to thrive 183, 185
   and fever 20
   history taking for 78–9
   and hypokalaemia 98
   and joint pain 206
   and palpitations 60
   and vaginal bleeding 159
   and vomiting 182
differential diagnosis
   in Calgary–Cambridge model
      1
   tips for 12
digoxin 216–17
disease framework, exploration
   of 3
disulfiram 146
diuretics 96, 98–9, 148–9, 170,
   208
diverticular disease 35, 80–1,
   84–5
diverticulitis 80, 82, 84
dizziness 60, 118–20, 131
DMARDs (disease modifying
   anti-rheumatic drugs) 209
domestic abuse 29
Doppler scan 23, 49
Down syndrome 42, 193
Duchenne's muscular dystrophy
   192–4
DVT (deep vein thrombosis)
   20, 48
dysarthria 71
dyschezia 93–4
dysmenorrhoea 92, 94
dyspareunia
   and dysuria 93–4
   in gynaecological history 154
   and subfertility 167
   and vaginal bleeding 156
   and vaginal discharge 163
dysphagia
   and breathlessness 58
   and cough 197
   differential diagnosis for 71–2
   and haemoptysis 67
   history taking for 70–1
   management of 73
   and motor neurone disease
      112
dyspnoea
   and breathlessness 57
   and claudication 48
   and epiglottitis 197
   exertional 58, 65
   and falls 104
   and motor neurone disease
      112
dysuria
   and cystitis 90, 97
   differential diagnosis for 93–4
   history taking for 92–3
   management of 94–5
   and vaginal discharge 163

eating disorders 76, 147–8, 173
EBV (Epstein–Barr virus) 43, 46
echocardiography 23, 58, 62, 104,
   146, 219
ectopic beats 61–2
eczema 24–5, 56–7, 65, 196
Ehlers–Danlos syndrome 30,
   54, 108
endocarditis, infectious 22–3, 67
endometrial cancer 157–8
endometriosis 94, 168, 204
epiglottitis 197
epilepsy 102, 188–90, 193
episcleritis 214
Epstein–Barr virus 17
examiners, friendliness to 8
expression, facial 2
eye pain 106, 114, 118, 213

facial nerve palsy 120, 123
facilitative response 2
failure to thrive 183–6
falls
   differential diagnosis of 103–4
   and forgetfulness 136, 138
   history taking for 102–3
   management of 104–5
familial Mediterranean fever 22
feeding history 178–9
   and failure to thrive 183
fever
   and alcohol withdrawal 132
   and back pain 204
   and breathlessness 56–7
   and cellulitis 26
   and chest pain 54
   in children 182, 189, 197
   differential diagnosis for 21–2
   and dysuria 90, 92–3, 97
   and haemoptysis 67–8
   and headache 106, 108
   history taking for 20–1
   and incontinence 169
   investigations for 23
   and red eye 212
   and tonsillitis 72
fibromyalgia 16, 18, 204, 208–9
finasteride 95, 98, 171
flatulence 78–9
flights, long-haul 52, 54, 57, 66
floaters 216, 218
fontanelle, bulging 182, 190
foreign bodies
   and hearing loss 121
   inhaled 64, 67, 197
   and red eye 213–14
   and vaginal discharge 165
forgetfulness 136–7, 139
friends, practising with 7
furosemide 59, 91

galactorrhoea 174
gallstones 35, 37, 45–6
ganglions 38, 40, 120

gastric carcinoma 74, 76
gastric erosions 75
gastroenteritis 80–1, 84–5, 94,
   182
genetic counselling 113
genital tract malignancy 165
genital warts 165
genitourinary prolapse 97–8
gentamicin 23, 119, 122, 124
Gilbert's syndrome 45
Glasgow–Blatchford score 76
glaucoma 107, 109, 212–14,
   217–19
globus pharyngeus 72–3
glomerulonephritis 88, 90–1
glue ear 122, 124
goitre 132, 142, 174
gonorrhoea 94, 165, 168
Goodpasture's syndrome 90
GORD (gastro-oesophageal
   reflux disease)
   and abdominal pain 35
   and chest pain 52, 54
   in children 181–2, 185
   and cough 64–5
   and dysphagia 70–2
Gottron's papules 111
gout 207–9
grandiosity 128, 135, 140–2
GTN (gliceryl trinitrate) 54, 59,
   85
gynaecological history 92, 96–7,
   154

haematemesis
   and abdominal pain 35
   differential diagnosis for 75–6
   and dysphagia 70–1
   history taking for 74–5
   management of 76–7
   and rectal bleeding 82, 84
haematuria
   differential diagnosis of 89–90
   and dysuria 94
   and fever 22
   history taking for 88–9
   and incontinence 169, 171
   management of 90–1
   and polyuria 96
haemolysis 46
haemophilia 29, 31, 90
haemoptysis
   and breathlessness 57–8
   and cancer 18, 22
   and chest pain 54
   and cough 64–5
   differential diagnosis for 67–8
   and fever 21
   and haematemesis 75
   and haematuria 90
   history taking for 66–7
haemorrhage
   antepartum 160–2
   intracranial 107–9, 120, 213

subconjunctival 214
  vitreal 218
haemorrhoids 82–3, 85
hair thinning 24, 61, 126, 174
halitosis 70, 72
hallucinations 128, 132–5, 138,
  142
haloes 212, 214, 218
hand dominance 193
hand washing 8
hay fever 25, 56–7, 65, 196, 213
headache
  and bruising 28
  and cough 63
  differential diagnosis of 107–9
  and dizziness 118
  and fever 20
  and glaucoma 214
  and hearing loss 121, 123
  history taking for 106–7
  and numbness 114
  and rash 24
  and seizures 103
  sentinel 106, 108
  and tiredness 16, 18
  and visual loss 216
  and weakness 110
  and weight loss 41
hearing loss 121–4
heart attacks, *see* myocardial
  infarction
heart disease
  and alcohol 146
  and breathlessness 56, 58
  and chest pain 53
  and palpitations 60
heart failure 18–19, 53, 58, 61, 66
heartburn
  and abdominal pain 34
  and cough 63
  and dysphagia 70, 72
  and haematemesis 75
  and lumps 38
  and rectal bleeding 82
  and weight loss 41
Helicobacter pylori 77
Henoch–Schönlein purpura 26,
  30
heparin 55, 59
hepatitis, and jaundice 45–6
hepatocellular carcinoma 46
hernias 38–40
herpes, genital 165
Herpes simplex 214–15
Herpes zoster 26–7, 36, 120,
  214–15
hirsutism 174–5
HIS MMM mnemonic 121, 123
history taking
  alternative structures for
    14–15
  similarity to real life 1
  structured framework for 5–6
  tips for 11–12

HIV 21, 43, 165
hoarse voice 58, 64, 67, 71
hot flushes 131, 172, 174
HPV (human papillomavirus)
  158, 164
HRT (hormone replacement
  therapy) 154–6, 159, 175
hyperbilirubinaemia 45
hypercalcaemia 98–9, 138
hypercholesterolaemia 47–8, 53
hyperparathyroidism 98
hyperprolactinaemia 168, 172,
  174–5
hypertension
  and antepartum haemorrhage
    160
  and anxiety 130
  and breathlessness 56
  and chest pain 52–3
  and claudication 47–8
  and falls 103
  and gout 208
  and haematuria 88, 91
  and incontinence 170
  and stroke 71
  and visual loss 216
hyperthyroidism
  and amenorrhoea 174–5
  and anxiety 129–32
  in children 185
  and weight loss 43
hyperventilation 109, 116
hypoglycaemia 132, 138, 190, 194
hypogonadism 168, 172, 174–5
hypokalaemia 98–9
hypomania 142
hypotension, postural 103–4
hypothyroidism
  and amenorrhoea 174–5
  in children 185
  and depression 126–8
  management of 19
  and thyroxine 4
  and tiredness 16–18

IBD (inflammatory bowel
  disease)
  and abdominal pain 35–6
  and bowel habit 78–81
  in children 181
  and joint pain 206
  and rectal bleeding 82–5
  and red eye 212, 214
  and weight loss 42–3
IBS (irritable bowel syndrome)
  16, 18, 35, 80, 208
icebreakers 8
ideas, flight of 140–1
IHD (ischaemic heart disease) 35,
  53, 58, 61, 216
ILL BUGS mnemonic 180
illness framework, incorporating
  4
immobilisation 48, 67

immune thrombocytopaenic
  purpura 31
immunisation history 178
immunosuppression 68, 113, 208
incontinence
  and back pain 204
  and convulsions 187
  and falls 102–3
  and haematuria 88
  and numbness 114
  and polyuria 96
  urinary 158, 169–71, 189
  and weakness 110
infections, screening questions
  for 20
infliximab 81, 85
information gathering 3–5
insomnia 142
insulin
  clues to use of 8
  and palpitations 60
  and tiredness 18–19
interviews, adapting 1
intracranial pressure, raised
  107–9, 115, 119, 182
intrauterine growth restriction
  184
intravenous drugs 21
intussusception 181–2
investigations 12

jargon 3
jaundice 5, 30, 44–5, 171
joint pain 22, 30, 206–9, 212

keratitis 213–14
kidney failure 18–19

labyrinthitis, acute 119–20
Lambert–Eaton myasthenic
  syndrome 112
language, appropriate use of 3
language therapy 73, 113, 194,
  200
laxatives 79, 81–2, 85, 98, 147–9
leg pain 5
legs, swollen 67
leukotriene antagonists 65, 197
Lewy bodies 137
libido 126–7, 140, 172, 174
limb ischaemia 48, 54
limb weakness 71, 112
lipomas 38–40
lithium 142
liver disease 18, 29–30, 74–5,
  145–6
liver failure 18–19, 138
low mood 16, 18, 126–7, 135, 142
LSD 135, 142
lumbar spondylosis 203
lumps
  and bruising 28
  differential diagnosis for 39–40
  and dysphagia 70

lumps (*continued*)
 and fever 20
 and haemoptysis 66
 history taking for 38–9
 and tiredness 16
lung abscess 67–8
lung cancer 19, 58, 63–8
lung disease, interstitial 58, 111, 208
lupus 24, 116, 160, 209
lymphadenopathy 21, 28–9, 66, 68

macroprolactinomas 174
macular degeneration 219
malabsorption
 and bowel habit 80–1
 and bruising 30
 in children 185
 and cystic fibrosis 196
 and weight loss 41–2
malaise
 and breathlessness 57
 and bronchitis 67
 and cough 63
 and endocarditis 22
 and haemoptysis 68
 and pneumonia 54
 and rash 26
malignancy
 and back pain 204
 and fever 22
 and lumps 39
 management of 23
 and PE 54, 57, 67
 and rectal bleeding 82–3
 screening questions for 20
 and weight loss 43
Mallory–Weiss tear 75–6
malnutrition 71
management, tips for 12
mania 126–8, 133, 135, 140–3
marasmus 41
Marfan's syndrome 30, 54, 57
meconium ileus 195–6
medications
 and fever 22
 and tiredness 18
melaena
 and abdominal pain 35
 in ALARMS symptoms 74, 76
 and dysphagia 71
 and fever 22
 and rectal bleeding 83
memory, short-term 136–8
Ménière's disease 119–20, 123–4
meningism 106
meningitis
 and bruising 28
 in children 182, 188, 190, 192
 and headache 107–9
 screening questions for 20, 24
meningococcal septicaemia 26–7, 108, 190

menopause
 and hearing loss 123
 premature 168, 174, 204
 signs of 174
 and urination 92, 96–7, 169
menorrhagia 16–17, 154, 174
menstrual history 154, 156, 163, 166, 172
menstrual irregularities
 and depression 126
 and palpitations 61
 and subfertility 166
 and tiredness 18
menstrual pain 35
meralgia paraesthetica 116
metamorphopsia 219
metformin 49, 98, 175
methylphenidate 200
migraine 106–7, 109, 120
miscarriages 158, 160–1, 166
MONAC 55, 59
Mongolian blue spot 30
mononeuritis multiplex 112, 116
mononucleosis, infectious 17, 19
morphine 55, 59, 135, 138
motor development, delay in 193
motor neurone disease 71, 112–13
mouth, dry 20, 22, 62, 129, 131, 206
mouth ulcers 78, 80, 82, 84, 206
multiple endocrine neoplasia 62
multiple sclerosis
 and dizziness 120
 and dysphagia 70
 and hearing loss 123
 and incontinence 170–1
 and numbness 117
 and visual loss 219
 and weakness 112
 and weight loss 43
mumps 121, 167–8
muscle haematomas 29, 36
muscle wasting 110–11
muscle weakness 98, 111, 169
muscular dystrophy 111, 113
musculoskeletal pain 18, 53–4
myalgia 18, 103, 111, 204, 208
myasthenia gravis 71, 111–13
myeloma, multiple 204
myocardial infarction 47–8, 54, 104–5
myopia 218

naltrexone 146
nasopharyngeal tumour 123
neck lumps 38–40
Neisseria gonorrhoeae 165
nephrotic syndrome 90–1
neurofibromatosis 38–9, 119
neuropathy, peripheral 112, 116–17
nitrates 55, 59
nocturia 88, 92–4, 96–8, 169

nosebleeds 28, 66–7, 75, 123
NSAIDs (non-steroidal anti-inflammatory drugs)
 and abdominal pain 35
 and back pain 205
 and dysphagia 70
 and haematemesis 74–5, 77
 and self-harm 151
 and spondyloarthropathy 209
 and tiredness 17
numbness
 and anxiety 131
 and claudication 48
 differential diagnosis of 115–16
 facial 123
 history taking for 114–15
 investigations for 117
 and rash 24
 and self-harm 151
 and weakness 110, 112–13
nyctalopia 219

O CAT RIB mnemonic 74
obesity
 and arthritis 208
 and bowel habit 80
 and haemoptysis 67
 and oligomenorrhoea 174
 and rectal bleeding 84
 and stroke 71
obsessive–compulsive disorder 129
occupational therapy 113, 200
odynophagia 72
oesophageal cancer 72
oesophageal stricture, benign 71, 73
oesophageal varices 75
oesophageal web 72
oesophagitis 75
oligomenorrhoea 128, 132, 172–4
ophthalmoscopy 109, 219
opioids 79
oppositional defiant disorder 200
optic neuritis 115, 218–19
orthopnoea 52–3, 58
OSCEs
 description of 1
 feasible performance in 4
 general tips for 7–9
OSLER 5
osteoarthritis 39, 48, 208–9
osteoporosis 104, 202–5
otitis media 122, 194, 197
otosclerosis 123–4
ototoxicity 119
ovarian cancer 79, 83, 157
ovarian cysts 168, 175

paediatric history 178–9
Paget's disease 98
pain, in history taking 5, 14
pallor 103, 182, 189

palpitations
  and anxiety 131–2
  and breathlessness 56
  and chest pain 52
  differential diagnosis of 61–2
  history taking for 60–1
pancreatitis 35, 45, 80, 204
panic 8, 60, 62, 129, 131
paracetamol 151, 190, 197
paraesthesia 115, 189, 203, 218
paraneoplastic syndrome 58, 64, 67, 89, 112
Parkinsonism 136
Parkinson's disease 97, 138, 170–1
paroxysmal nocturnal dyspnoea 52–3, 58
patients
  friendliness to 8
  unreliability of 4
patient's perspective 3, 5, 11
PCI (percutaneous coronary intervention) 55, 59
pelvic inflammatory disease 165, 168
peptic ulcers 35–6, 74–5, 82, 84
perception, delusions of 134, 142
pericarditis 53–4
peritonitis 75
pertussis 197
pessaries 95, 98
pets 196
phaeochromocytoma 60, 62, 132
pharyngeal pouch 72
pharyngitis 72
phobias 129, 131
photophobia 107–8, 214
placenta praevia 161–2
Plummer–Vinson syndrome 72
pneumonia
  and atrial fibrillation 61
  and breathlessness 57, 59
  and chest pain 53–4
  in children 197
  and cough 64
  and dysphagia 71
  and haemoptysis 68
  management of 59, 65, 68
  streptococcal 43
polycystic kidney disease 38–40, 89, 106–8
polycystic ovarian syndrome 158, 166–8, 172–5
polydipsia 18, 97–8
polymyalgia rheumatica 22–3, 106
polymyositis 111, 113
polyneuropathy 116
polyps, cervical 158, 162
polyuria 18, 96–9
post-ictal state 102–3, 187, 190
post-nasal drip 64–5
post-traumatic stress disorder 131

Pott's disease 204
pre-eclampsia 178
pre-syncope 119
prednisolone 109, 113
pregnancy
  and amenorrhoea 174
  and candidiasis 165
  and DVT 48
  ectopic 37, 157–9
  and hearing loss 123
  maternal illnesses during 178
  and PE 54, 57, 67
  and vaginal bleeding 158
premature ejaculation 167
professionalism 8
prolapse, and urination 96, 169
prolapsed intervertebral disc 203, 205
propranolol 62, 175
props 2, 8, 56
prostate, resection of 95, 168, 171
prostate cancer 18, 90, 171
prostatitis 90, 92–3, 96
proton-pump inhibitors 65, 77
pruritis
  and jaundice 44
  and red eye 212–13
pruritis ani 83
psoriasis 24–5, 27, 206–7, 214
psychosis 126, 135–6, 140–2, 144
ptosis 71
pulmonary embolism (PE) 53–5, 57, 59, 66–8
pulmonary oedema 58–9
pulmonary rehabilitation 58
purpuric rash 26–7
pyelonephritis 93–4
pyloric stenosis 181–2

radioiodine 62, 175
radiotherapy 23, 65, 68, 120, 171, 205
Ramsay Hunt syndrome 120
rashes
  differential diagnosis for 25–6
  and fever 20, 22
  history taking for 24–5
  macular 111
  management of 27
  and meningitis 182
  and red eye 212
  and SLE 208
Raynaud's phenomenon
  and dysphagia 72
  and fever 22
  and numbness 116
  and SLE 208
  and weakness 111
reading time 7
recreational drugs
  and abdominal pain 35
  and alcohol 145
  and antepartum haemorrhage 161

  and anxiety 130
  and bruising 29
  and depression 127
  and dizziness 119
  and haematemesis 75
  and headache 107
  history taking for 103
  and jaundice 45
  and mania 141
  and numbness 115
  and palpitations 61
  in pregnancy 184, 187
  and self-harm 151
  and subfertility 167
  and tiredness 17
  and vaginal discharge 164
  and visual loss 217
  and weakness 111
  and weight loss 42
rectal bleeding 80, 82–5, 182
red eye 78, 82, 109, 206, 212–15
red-flag symptoms
  and abdominal pain 35
  and back pain **203**, 205
  and diarrhoea 79
  and headache 107
  and rectal bleeding 83
  and red eye 213
referred pain 36, 213
rehydration 81, 85, 182
Reiter's syndrome 94, 214
renal calculi 90, 93–5, 204
renal cell carcinoma 89–90
renal failure
  and bruising 30
  in children 185
  and claudication 49
  and gout 208
  and haematuria 88
  and tiredness 19
retinal artery occlusion 217, 219
retinal detatchment 218–19
retinitis pigmentosa 217, 219
retrograde ejaculation 168
rheumatoid arthritis
  and fever 22
  and joint pain 207–8
  and lumps 39
  management of 23, 209
  and red eye 212
  and scleritis 214
  and weight loss 43
rickets 194
risk assessment, for self-harm and suicide 126, 128, 133–4, 136, 150
rivastigmine 138
Rockall score 76

salbutamol PRN 65, 197
scalp tenderness 109, 217
schistosomiasis 89
schizoaffective disorder 128, 142
schizophrenia 126–7, 134–5, 142

Schneider's first-rank symptoms 134, 142
sciatica 48
scleritis 213–14
SCOFF questions 147
seizures
　and alcohol withdrawl 132
　and dizziness 118
　and falls 102–3, 105
　and headache 106
　and meningitis 108
　reflex anoxic 189–90
　and weakness 110
self-esteem 135, 140–1, 152
self-harm 126, 129, 134, 140, 145, 150–2
senile purpura 30
septic arthritis 207–9
sexual abuse 131, 151
sexual disinhibition 136, 141
sexual history 92–3, 155–6, 163–4
sexual orientation 164
shingles 26, 116
shortness of breath
　and anxiety 131
　and breathlessness 57
　and chest pain 54
　and fever 20, 22
　and haemoptysis 67–8
　and myasthenia gravis 71
SIADH (syndrome of inappropriate antidiuretic hormone secretion) 58, 64, 67
signposting 3, 9, 126
simulated patients (SPs)
　help from 11
　in history taking 1
　and professionalism 8
sinusitis 64, 108
skin
　thin 67
　tight 70, 72
skin lesions 20, 22
SLE (systemic lupus erythematosus) 22–3, 43, 167, 208, 214
sleep
　and depression 126
　and mania 140
　and tiredness 16
sleep hygiene 19, 128
smoking
　and antepartum haemorrhage 161
　and breathlessness 57–8
　and cervical cancer 158, 162
　and claudication 47, 49
　and cough 64–5
　and dizziness 119–20
　effects on children 183, 187, 191, 195–6
　and forgetfulness 138
　and hearing loss 122–4

and pain 14
and subfertility 167–8
smoking and jaundice 45
social impairment 198, 200
social isolation 134, 142
social phobia 131
SOCRATES mnemonic, alternatives to 14–15
sore throat
　and cough 64, 195, 197
　and tiredness 16–18
speech, picking up cues from 2
speech development, delayed 194
spinal canal stenosis 204
spinal claudication 48
spinal cord
　compression 202–3, 205
　lesion 78
spinal stenosis 112, 116
splenectomy 27, 31
spondyloarthropathy 204, 206–7, 209, 214
spondylolisthesis 116
spotter stations 7
SSRIs
　and anxiety 132
　and depression 128
　and eating disorders 149
　and haematemesis 75, 77
　and palpitations 62
　and tiredness 19
Staphylococcus aureus 27
statins 47, 49, 55, 59
steatorrhoea 30, 80, 182, 196
steroids
　and abdominal pain 35
　and breathlessness 58–9
　and bruising 29
　and cough 65
　and dysphagia 70
　and haematemesis 74, 77
　and hallucinations 135
　and lupus 209
　and numbness 117
　and rectal bleeding 85
　and red eye 213, 215
　and visual loss 219
　and weakness 113
STIs (sexually transmitted infections)
　and cervical cancer 162
　and dysuria 93
　and fever 20
　and rash 206
　and red eye 212
　and subfertility 166–7
　and vaginal bleeding 157, 159
　and vaginal discharge 164–5
Stokes–Adams attack 104
STOP mnemonic 70
stress
　acute reaction to 131
　and amenorrhoea 174
　and bowel habit 80

and haematemesis 75
and hallucinations 133
and headache 108
and numbness 114
and polyuria 97
stridor 58, 64, 67, 197
stroke
　and claudication 47–8
　and dizziness 120
　and dysphagia 70–1
　and hallucinations 135
　and hearing loss 123
　and numbness 115, 117
　and palpitations 62
　and weakness 112
subfertility 94, 154, 165–7, 174
suicide 127–8, 134, 151–2
sulfasalazine 23, 81, 85
summarising 3–4, 11–12
support groups 146
surgical sieves 42, 123
swallowing, pain in 70–1
sweating
　and ACS 57
　and anxiety 116, 129, 131–2
　and chest pain 52
　and menopause 172, 174
　and myocardial infarction 104
　and weight loss 41
swelling 26, 38, 206–8
symptom analysis 3, 178
syncope 61, 103–4, 190
syphilis 121, 135, 138, 165, 214
syringomyelia 112, 116
systemic sclerosis 72–3
systems review
　and abdominal pain 34
　in Calgary–Cambridge model 3
　and lumps 38–9
　tips for 11

tachycardia 26, 61–2, 67, 116
tamsulosin 95, 98, 171
temporal arteritis
　and fever 20, 22–3
　and headache 106–7, 109
　and visual loss 216–17, 219
tension headaches 107–8
tension pneumothorax 54–5, 57
testicular torsion 37, 167–8
thiamine, *see* vitamin B$_1$
thiazides 207
thigh numbness 116
thrombocytopaenia 29
thrombolysis 55, 59, 117
thyroid disease
　and amenorrhoea 173
　and depression 126
　and fever 21
　and forgetfulness 138
　and mania 141
　and subfertility 168
　and tiredness 16–18
thyroidectomy 62

thyrotoxicosis 42, 60–2
thyroxine 4, 19, 60, 175
TIA (transient ischaemic attack) 115, 120
time framing 2
tinnitus 119–20, 122–3
tiredness 16–19, 82
Todd's paralysis 102
tongue-biting 102–3, 187, 189–90
tonometry 214, 219
tonsillitis 72, 197
Tourette's syndrome 200
toxic shock syndrome 163, 165
transitional cell carcinoma 89
tremor
    and anxiety 129, 131–2
    and forgetfulness 136–7
    and phaeochromocytoma 62
    and thyrotoxicosis 61
Trichomonas vaginalis 164–5
tricyclic antidepressants 104
trigeminal neuralgia 109
trimethoprim 91, 94, 98
triptans 109
tuberculosis (TB)
    and back pain 202, 204
    and fever 21, 23
    and haemoptysis 68
    and weight loss 43
tuberous sclerosis 188, 190, 193
tunnel vision 216
Turner's syndrome 173
tympanic membrane perforation 122, 124

ulcerative colitis 79, 81, 85
understanding, shared 4
urethritis 93–4
urinalysis 19, 23, 37, 43, 90, 185
urination
    and falls 104
    pain in 93
    problems with 16
URTI (upper respiratory tract infection)
    and bruising 30
    and cough 63–4, 195, 197
    and failure to thrive 185
    and fever 20
    and haematuria 90
    and rash 24
urticaria 22, 26
UTI (urinary tract infections)
    and abdominal pain 35
    and dysuria 93–4
    and fever 20

and haematuria 88, 90–1
and hallucinations 135
and polyuria 97–8
and rash 24
recurrent 97, 158
uveitis 206, 213–15

vaginal atrophy 174–5
vaginal bleeding 154, 156–9
vaginal discharge 92, 154, 163–5
vaginal prolapse 170
vaginismus 168
vaginitis, atrophic 94–5, 158–9
vaginosis, bacterial 165
Valsalva manoeuvre 62, 108
valvular disease 22, 61
Varicella zoster 26, 120
varicocoeles 168
varicose veins 39
vascular dementia 137
vascular disease 47–8, 137, 216
vasculitis 20, 22–3, 43, 90, 123, 214
venous sinus thrombosis 107
vertigo 119–23
viral illness
    and rashes 26
    and tiredness 16–17
vision, blurred 214, 216–19
visual aids 3
vitamin A 219
vitamin B_1 146
vitamin B_{12} 17, 135, 138, 217
vitamin D 205
vitamin K 30–1
vomit, coffee-ground 75
vomiting
    and abdominal pain 34, 37
    and bowel habit 78, 80
    and breathlessness 57
    and bruising 29
    and chest pain 53
    and cough 197
    and dizziness 119
    and fever 20
    and glaucoma 214
    and haematemesis 74, 76
    and haemoptysis 66
    and headache 106
    and hypercalcaemia 98
    and incontinence 171
    induced 147
    and lumps 38
    paediatric 180–3
    and rectal bleeding 84
    and red eye 212, 214

and vaginal bleeding 159
and weight loss 41
von Willebrand's disease 29

WAIF questions 147
warfarin
    and breathlessness 59
    and bruising 28–9
    and claudication 47
    and haematemesis 74
    and haemoptysis 66
    and palpitations 62
    and PE 55
water tablets 148, 170
weakness
    and bowel habit 78
    differential diagnosis of 111–12
    and dizziness 118
    and dysphagia 70–1
    and falls 102
    history taking for 110–11
    and hypokalaemia 98
    management of 113
weight loss
    and abdominal pain 34–5
    and alcohol 144
    and back pain 202–4
    and breathlessness 56, 58
    and bruising 28
    and cervical cancer 162
    and cough 63–4
    and depression 127
    and diabetes 97
    differential diagnosis for 42–3
    and dysphagia 70–1
    and fever 21–2
    and haemoptysis 66–8
    and hearing loss 121
    history taking for 41–2
    and incontinence 169, 171
    and lumps 38–9
    and polyuria 96
    and rectal bleeding 82
    and tiredness 18
    and vaginal bleeding 157
    and vitamin K deficiency 30
Wernicke's encephalopathy 146
wheeze
    and breathlessness 56–8
    and cough 63–4
    and haemoptysis 67
Wolff–Parkinson–White syndrome 61

xerophthalmia 212